Bacterial Sexually Transmitted Infections - New Findings, Diagnosis, Treatment, and Prevention

Edited by Mihaela Laura Vică

Published in London, United Kingdom

Bacterial Sexually Transmitted Infections - New Findings, Diagnosis, Treatment, and Prevention
http://dx.doi.org/10.5772/intechopen.100799
Edited by Mihaela Laura Vică

Contributors
Lebeza Alemu Tenaw, Susu M. Zughaier, Emna Rigane, Simeon Chijioke Amadi, Joseph Okoeguale, Williams Amebeobari Mube, Anthony Chukwuemeka Olobuah, Chibuzor Peter Oriji, Irina Khamaganova, Nikolay Potekaev, Olga Zhukova, Diana Leticia Coronel Martínez, Luis Augusto Moya-Barquín, Mihaela Laura Vică

First published in London, United Kingdom, 2023 by IntechOpen
IntechOpen is the global imprint of INTECHOPEN LIMITED, registered in England and Wales, registration number: 11086078, 5 Princes Gate Court, London, SW7 2QJ, United Kingdom
Printed in Croatia

British Library Cataloguing-in-Publication Data
A catalogue record for this book is available from the British Library

Additional hard and PDF copies can be obtained from orders@intechopen.com

Bacterial Sexually Transmitted Infections - New Findings, Diagnosis, Treatment, and Prevention
Edited by Mihaela Laura Vică
p. cm.

This title is part of the Infectious Diseases Book Series, Volume 21
Topic: Bacterial Infectious Diseases
Series Editor: Alfonso J. Rodriguez-Morales
Topic Editors: Tomas Jarzembowski and Katarzyna Garbacz

Print ISBN 978-1-80356-749-5
Online ISBN 978-1-80356-750-1
eBook (PDF) ISBN 978-1-80356-751-8
ISSN 2631-6188

IntechOpen Book Series

Infectious Diseases

Volume 21

Aims and Scope of the Series

This series will provide a comprehensive overview of recent research trends in various Infectious Diseases (as per the most recent Baltimore classification). Topics will include general overviews of infections, immunopathology, diagnosis, treatment, epidemiology, etiology, and current clinical recommendations for managing infectious diseases. Ongoing issues, recent advances, and future diagnostic approaches and therapeutic strategies will also be discussed. This book series will focus on various aspects and properties of infectious diseases whose deep understanding is essential for safeguarding the human race from losing resources and economies due to pathogens.

Meet the Series Editor

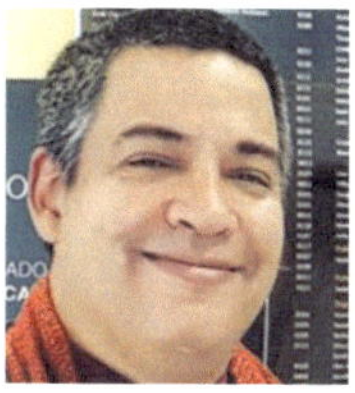

Dr. Rodriguez-Morales is an expert in tropical and emerging diseases, particularly zoonotic and vector-borne diseases (notably arboviral diseases), and more recently COVID-19 and Monkeypox. He is the president of the Publications and Research Committee of the Pan-American Infectious Diseases Association (API), as well as the president of the Colombian Association of Infectious Diseases (ACIN). He is a member of the Committee on Tropical Medicine, Zoonoses, and Travel Medicine of ACIN. Dr. Rodriguez-Morales is a vice-president of the Latin American Society for Travel Medicine (SLAMVI) and a member of the Council of the International Society for Infectious Diseases (ISID). Since 2014, he has been recognized as a senior researcher at the Ministry of Science of Colombia. He is a professor at the Faculty of Medicine of the Fundacion Universitaria Autonoma de las Americas, in Pereira, Risaralda, Colombia, and a professor, Master in Clinical Epidemiology and Biostatistics, at Universidad Científica del Sur, Lima, Peru. He is also a non-resident adjunct faculty member at the Gilbert and Rose-Marie Chagoury School of Medicine, Lebanese American University, Beirut, Lebanon, and an external professor, Master in Research on Tropical Medicine and International Health, at Universitat de Barcelona, Spain. Additionally, an invited professor, Master in Biomedicine, at Universidad Internacional SEK, Quito, Ecuador, and a visiting professor, Master Program of Epidemiology, at Diponegoro University, Indonesia. In 2021 he was awarded the "Raul Isturiz Award" Medal of the API and, the same year, the "Jose Felix Patiño" Asclepius Staff Medal of the Colombian Medical College due to his scientific contributions to the topic of COVID-19 during the pandemic. He is currently the Editor in Chief of the journal Travel Medicine and Infectious Diseases. His Scopus H index is 55 (Google Scholar H index 77) with a total of 725 publications indexed in Scopus.

Meet the Volume Editor

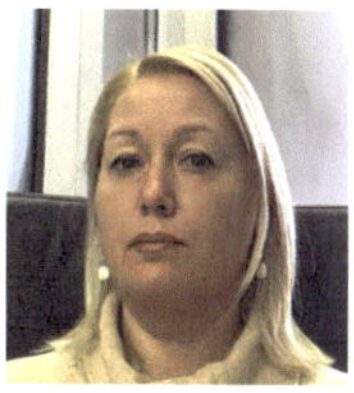

Dr. Mihaela Laura Vică, MSc, Ph.D., is an associate professor in the Cell and Molecular Biology Department, "Iuliu Hațieganu" University of Medicine and Pharmacy, Romania, where she obtained her Ph.D. in Medicine. She obtained her MSc in Cellular Biology from the Faculty of Biology, "Babeş-Bolyai" University, Romania. Since 2006, Dr. Vică has been involved in scientific research activities, coordinating an international cooperation research project and participating in more than thirty national and international conferences where she received five awards. She has published two books, two book chapters, and more than fifty research papers in international journals. Her areas of research are microbiology and molecular biology.

Contents

Preface

Sexually transmitted infections (STIs) are commonly caused by bacteria, viruses, or parasites transmitted in different ways such as vaginal, anal, and oral sexual contact. They can also be transmitted from pregnant persons to their fetuses during pregnancy or during birth. STIs are some of the most serious infections, as asymptomatic and untreated STIs lead to long-term health problems such as infertility. Despite worldwide efforts and precautions, STIs remain a serious public health problem.

Many STIs are caused by bacterial infectious agents. These infections are considered treatable, but, if they are not diagnosed or are diagnosed too late, they can seriously affect the health of those infected.

Bacterial Sexually Transmitted Infections - New Findings, Diagnosis, Treatment, and Prevention provides current information on some aspects of these infections in different regions of the world. The chapters are authored by known experts in the field who collaborated to provide valuable information on bacterial STIs from their own experience as well as from the specialized literature.

The book discusses various aspects of bacterial STIs, such as incidence in certain regions, impact on vulnerable categories, detection methods, and problems encountered during diagnosis and treatment. It begins with a chapter that introduces the specifics of the book, addressing the latest trends regarding the approach to bacterial STIs. The next two chapters present the most common bacterial STIs, highlighting their clinical manifestations, diagnosis, treatment, and prevention, and their impact on the general population as well as children. After that there is a chapter on the diagnosis of syphilis and the problems that may appear in the case of false-positive reactions, with examples from the author's own experience. The final two chapters examine the treatment of bacterial STIs, one showing the difficulties encountered in resource-limited settings, and the other presenting a new therapeutic target as an alternative for the treatment of gonorrhea, which is a widespread STI.

I would like to thank all the authors for their contributions and the time spent preparing this valuable collection. I would also like to extend my thanks to the staff at IntechOpen, particularly Ms. Marica Novaković for her great help during the editing of this book.

Mihaela Laura Vică, MSc, Ph.D.
Cell and Molecular Biology Department,
"Iuliu Hațieganu" University of Medicine and Pharmacy,
Cluj-Napoca, Romania

Chapter 1

Introductory Chapter: Bacterial Sexually Transmitted Infections – New Perspectives

Mihaela Laura Vică

1. Introduction

Sexually transmitted infections (STIs) are some of the most common infections worldwide. Newer sexually transmitted pathogens have been recognized and functionally described since 1980, with over 30 such infectious products currently known, which may be bacteria, viruses, or parasites. Today, conditions exist in developing countries that lead to an ever-increasing rate of STIs. Factors that influence this growth are: population explosion, especially in age groups that include teenagers and young people, population migration to urban areas, wars, or poverty. In these countries, in addition to human immunodeficiency virus (HIV) infection, three sexually transmitted bacterial infections (gonorrhea, chlamydia, and syphilis) can be considered among the first to affect the health of the population and reproductive life.

The most common sexually transmitted infection worldwide is chlamydia, with approximately 146 million infections each year. But while trends in increasing numbers of *Chlamydia* spp. infections appear to have stabilized in recent years, gonorrhea rates have increased, especially among men. The 2013 report on STIs in Europe shows that, in the countries of the European Union and the European Economic Area, STIs differ by age group: young adults between 15 and 25 had only 14% of syphilis cases but had nearly 39% of gonorrhea and 67% of chlamydia cases [1].

The Centers for Diseases Control and Prevention's (CDC) estimates that the prevalence and cost of STIs in the United States indicate that 20% of the population in this region (about one in five people) had an STI in 2018, infections that have cost that year almost 16 billion dollars in direct medical costs from the budget of the American health system [2].

No STI can be viewed and treated as an isolated infection because multiple infections are very common and the presence of an STI denotes high-risk sexual behavior that may be associated with other infections, which may be more serious. STIs can be classified based on both cause and clinical manifestations. Some of the pathogens can also be transmitted non-sexually, but for each of them, sexual transmission is clinically and epidemiologically important.

Many STIs are caused by bacterial infectious agents. In general, most STIs caused by bacteria are treatable, but if they go undiagnosed or are diagnosed too late, they can seriously affect the health of infected people. Thus, early detection and treatment can reduce the spread of bacterial STIs in the population.

Bacterial vaginosis is known to be highly implicated in female infertility and is probably a major cause of unexplained infertility. Screening and treatment of bacterial vaginitis during infertility treatment has greatly decreased its rate [3].

2. The most common bacterial STI pathogens

Chlamydia trachomatis infections are the most reported STI worldwide. However, it is known that there are many infections caused by this bacterium that go undiagnosed and consequently remain untreated. *C. trachomatis* can persist for a long time in the genital tract in a resistant form, and symptoms of infection may go unnoticed in about 75–80% of women [4]. Since many cases are asymptomatic, the actual detection of the infection would require screening in the population [5]. It is very important to diagnose this bacterium in the early stages of infection and start treatment as quickly as possible to avoid complications that may occur in the long term, thus reducing the risk of reproductive tract sequelae.

Lymphogranuloma venereum (LGV) is a disease caused by *C. trachomatis* serotypes L1, L2, and L3. It is considered endemic to Asia, Africa, South America, and the southeastern United States. In Europe, LGV infection is found almost exclusively in men who have sex with men (MSM), presenting clinically as a proctocolitis commonly associated with HIV [6].

Neisseria gonorrhoeae is the etiological agent of gonorrhea, one of the most common bacterial STIs, which is characterized by purulent inflammation of the mucous membranes of the genitourinary system, producing over 82 million new infections worldwide every year. Since 2008, the total number of gonorrhea cases has increased by 79%, especially among men. This increase appears to be related to the increase in cases among MSM [1]. Being a bacterium with remarkable genetic variability has led to the emergence and spread of multidrug-resistant strains of *N. gonorrhoeae*. This antibiotic resistance and the absence of an effective vaccine are major problems worldwide, highlighting the need for routine surveillance, prevention, and control measures [7].

Treponema pallidum is the etiological agent of syphilis, one of the bacterial STIs known for centuries [8]. Syphilis is a disease characterized by a decades-long clinical course that may include four different stages, without adequate treatment leading to either death or spontaneous resolution after the secondary stage. The overall rate of syphilis has increased since 2010, especially among men. In Europe, the incidence of syphilis has been reported to be five times higher in men than in women, and most cases occur in people over 25 years of age [1]. It is a serious disease because treponemes can cross the hemato-encephalic barrier and trigger neurological signs and symptoms, the risk being higher in patients with immunodeficiency or HIV. Syphilis can be transmitted from mother to unborn child, the stage of the mother's disease during pregnancy has an important role. If the mother's infection is massive it will lead to spontaneous abortion, but if there are few pathogens in the mother's blood, the child will develop congenital syphilis [6]. The upward trend in syphilis rates in many EU countries may be partly explained by increased case finding due to more testing among HIV-positive MSM, as recommended in current HIV management guidelines, or by an improved and more efficient reporting of detected cases.

Mycoplasmas are the smallest free-living microorganisms that lack a cell wall. Genital mycoplasmas are represented by species frequently found in the lower genitourinary tract of sexually active people, the most widespread being *Mycoplasma hominis*, *Ureaplasma urealyticum,* and *Mycoplasma genitalium*. Data suggest that infection with *U. urealyticum* occurs in 10–50% of women and that with *M. hominis* in less than 20% of them [9]. Since they have a high prevalence among asymptomatic women, their role in sexually transmitted diseases should be well evaluated [10]. These species of microorganisms are considered to induce a wide spectrum of pathological conditions in the lower urinary tract and genital organs, and *M. genitalium* would be implicated as a causative agent in conditions with significant sequelae. Some studies have reported that these organisms are involved in female infertility or premature birth [11]. In addition, some studies present mycoplasmas as causative agents of male infertility by changing some sperm characteristics [12].

Klebsiella granulomatis (formerly known as *Calymmatobacterium granulomatis*) is a gram-negative bacterium, the causative agent of donovanosis, a chronic ulcerative genital disease. The disease rarely occurs in Western European countries but is common in parts of Africa and South America. Transmission is mostly sexual, so infection with this bacterium can be considered an STI.

3. Diagnosis of bacterial STIs

The bacteria that cause STIs are very different from each other, so the methods of detecting bacterial STIs are very varied. Even for the same bacteria, there are different test methods. Substantial differences between testing methods and surveillance systems in different countries mean that many infections go undiagnosed and thus go unreported.

For example, the laboratory diagnosis of syphilis is based primarily on a series of serological tests: a positive screening test followed by a confirmatory test. Since antibodies can only be detected about 3 weeks after infection, the very early stage of the disease cannot be diagnosed serologically. Dark-field microscopy is used for epithelial lesions, and nucleic acid amplification tests (NAATs) have recently been introduced that can be used for direct detection of the causative pathogen [6].

Also, for the detection of *C. trachomatis*, immunoglobulin antibodies (IgG) persist in the body for years and therefore can be used as markers for infection [13], but the presence of antibodies does not indicate an infection present in the body at the time of detection, so these markers cannot be used in diagnosis.

Although bacterial cultures are considered by some to be the gold standard, some of the bacteria that cause STIs are very difficult to grow on culture media, and therefore most clinicians are unable to correctly assess the presence of one or another STI agent, if use these microbiological methods. For example, *M. genitalium* is difficult to grow on culture media because it has slow growth, strict nutrient requirements, and suitable culture media is not widely available [14]. On the other hand, due to the difficulties of sample collection, transfer, and storage, these methods show low sensitivity and are not suitable for screening, as some bacteria are fragile and difficult to transport.

New laboratory methods using the Polymerase Chain Reaction (PCR) technique allow rapid and targeted detection of STI pathogens, and the multiplex real-time PCR (RT-PCR) technique can be successfully used for the detection of multiple agents from a single sample STI, considering their association in many cases. These genetic tests allow establishing a diagnosis in a maximum of 2–3 days, with a sensitivity of up to 99%. In contrast, cell cultures provide a sensitivity of 85–95% in acute urethral infections with *N. gonorrhoeae* and less than 50% in chronic forms in women [15].

These multiplex RT-PCR kits are suitable for the routine detection of these STIs. They have proven to be cost-effective and rapid diagnostic tools with high reliability for the simultaneous detection of multiple pathogens present [16].

4. Treatment of bacterial STIs and resistance to antibiotics

Since its introduction against syphilis, in 1943, penicillin has remained the treatment for this disease, at all stages, and until now, no forms of resistance have been reported [6].

With respect to *C. trachomatis*, infections unresponsive to tetracycline or doxycycline have been reported, but pathogenic strains of this bacterium showing stable resistance to tetracycline have not yet been isolated from humans [17]. However, in the case of chlamydiosis, it is very likely that the infections will reappear even if adequate treatment has been used. This fact is due to reinfection or relapse, if the bacteria deviate to persistent phenotypes, resistant to antibiotics [18].

The three classes of antibiotics used in the treatment of *Ureaplasma* spp. are quinolones, tetracyclines, and macrolides, tetracycline being the most frequently used drug in the treatment of *U. urealyticum* infections [19]. In bacteria, tetracycline resistance is encoded by several genetic determinants, of which *TetM* is the only tetracycline resistance determinant reported so far in mycoplasmas. Using NAATs, both the presence of mycoplasmas and their resistance to this antibiotic can be determined from a single biological product sample [20].

The biggest problems with antibiotic resistance occur with *N. gonorrhoeae*. Being a bacterium capable of incorporating and changing DNA, as well as transferring modified DNA sequences, *N. gonorrhoeae* is known as a bacterium that readily develops mutations. This fact is important both for the development of antibiotic resistance and also has an important role in developing the diagnosis using NAATs, considering that the sensitivity of a certain molecular test can be decreased if the target is a genetically modified region. In recent years, *N. gonorrhoeae* has become less sensitive to several antibiotics, such as sulfonamides, penicillin, tetracyclines, fluoroquinolones, and even cephalosporins, thus defending multiresistant strains to antibiotics and therefore the appropriate treatment is sometimes difficult to apply. In many countries, dual antimicrobial therapy (ceftriaxone plus azithromycin) is the recommended first-line empiric treatment [21]. Due to the phenomenon of resistance, lately, natural products are increasingly being sought as possible alternative treatments for gonorrhea [22].

Resistance of microorganisms to antibiotics is a very dynamic phenomenon, which highlights the need to update prevalence and susceptibility data in different geographical areas. The use of molecular tests for surveillance of antimicrobial resistance in sexually transmitted bacteria would provide a significant advantage in terms of public health and the treatment of these diseases [23].

5. Transmission and prevention

In recent years, the incidence of STIs seems to have decreased in industrialized countries that make sustained efforts to prevent and combat these infections, but it remains a big problem everywhere in the world, especially in developing countries. To prevent the spread of these infections, there are several approaches, such as: reducing the rate of changing partners, encouraging safer sexual practices, such as the use of condoms, detecting and treating them in early stages, or even introducing screening programs in the population groups with increased risk of contracting such infections. However, there are certain constraints that prevent the effective application of prevention methods such as: the lack of sexual education programs for children and young people, the available time of clinicians, and, finally, the financial aspects regarding the costs for the implementation of modern laboratory methods for accurate detection of the causative pathogen or determination of antibiotic resistance. As the prevalence of bacterial STIs is increasing in the MSM community, a recent pilot study demonstrated the effectiveness of reducing the transmission of these bacterial infections using pre-exposure prophylaxis by daily administration of doxycycline to men in this community [24].

Besides this, there are opinions that claim that vaccination against sexually transmitted pathogens would be indicated, especially in the case of *N. gonorrhoeae*. This approach can be successful if the origins of antibodies in the genital tract and the mechanisms by which they could exercise protective immunity are elucidated [25]. In recent years, progress has been made regarding the understanding of the molecular basis of the pathogenesis of the infection and the mechanisms of host cell damage, including those of escape from immune surveillance with the aim of obtaining effective vaccines against these bacteria.

Therefore, this book attempts a new approach regarding different aspects of bacterial STIs, presenting points of view, challenges, or individual research, to open new perspectives on this field in order to use advanced methods of diagnosis, treatment, control, and prevention of these infections that affect a large part of the population all over the world.

Author details

Mihaela Laura Vică
Department of Cell and Molecular Biology, "Iuliu Hațieganu" University of Medicine and Pharmacy, Cluj-Napoca, Romania

*Address all correspondence to: mvica@umfcluj.ro

References

[1] ECDC. Sexually transmitted infections in Europe. 2013. Available from: https://www.ecdc.europa.eu/en/publications-data/sexually-transmitted-infections-europe-2013. [Accessed: October 8, 2022]

[2] CDC. Incidence, prevalence, and cost of sexually transmitted infections in the United States. 2021. Available from: https://www.cdc.gov/nchhstp/newsroom/fact-sheets/std/sti-incidence-prevalence-cost-factsheet.html. [Accessed: October 8, 2022]

[3] Salah RM, Allam AM, Magdy AM, Mohamed AS. Bacterial vaginosis and infertility: Cause or association? European Journal of Obstetrics, Gynecology, and Reproductive Biology. 2013;**167**(1):59-63. DOI: 10.1016/j.ejogrb.2012.10.031

[4] Witkin SS, Linhares LM. Chlamydia trachomatis in subfertile women undergoing uterine instrumentation. Human Reproduction. 2002;**17**(8):525-527. DOI: 10.1093/humrep/17.3.525

[5] Geisler WM. Diagnosis and management of uncomplicated Chlamydia trachomatis infections in adolescents and adults: Summary of evidence reviewed for the 2015 centers for disease control and prevention sexually transmitted diseases treatment guidelines. Clinical Infectious Diseases. 2015;**61**:S774-S784. DOI: 10.1093/cid/civ694

[6] Buder S, Schöfer H, Meyer T, Bremer V, Kohl PK, Skaletz-Rorowski A, et al. Bacterial sexually transmitted infections. Journal der Deutschen Dermatologischen Gesellschaft. 2019;**17**(3):287-315. DOI: 10.1111/ddg.13804

[7] Bilek N, Martin IM, Bell G, Kinghorn GR, Ison CA, Spratt BG. Concordance between Neisseria gonorrhoeae genotypes recovered from known sexual contacts. Journal of Clinical Microbiology. 2007;**45**(11):3564-3567. DOI: 10.1128/JCM.01453-07

[8] Eickhoff CA, Decker CF. Syphilis. Disease-a-Month. 2016;**62**(8):280-286. DOI: 10.1016/j.disamonth.2016.03.012

[9] Daxboeck F, Iro E, Tamussino K, Krause R, Assadian O, Wenisch C. Bacteremia with Mycoplasma hominis and Ureaplasma urealyticum in patients undergoing hysterectomy. European Journal of Clinical Microbiology & Infectious Diseases. 2003;**22**(10):608-611. DOI: 10.1007/s10096-003-1001-8

[10] Peerayeh SN, Sattari M. Detection of Ureaplasma urealyticum and Mycoplasma hominis in endocervical specimens from infertile women by polymerase chain reaction. Middle East Fertility Society Journal. 2006;**11**(2):104-108

[11] Gupta A, Gupta A, Gupta S, Mittal A, Chandra P, Gill AK. Correlation of mycoplasma with unexplained infertility. Archives of Gynecology and Obstetrics. 2009;**280**(6):981-985. DOI: 10.1007/s00404-009-1042-z

[12] Reichart M, Kahane I, Bartoov B. In vivo and in vitro impairment of human and ram sperm nuclear chromatin integrity by sexually transmitted Ureaplasma urealyticum infection. Biology of Reproduction. 2000;**63**(4):1041-1048. DOI: 10.1095/biolreprod63.4.1041

[13] Mol BW, Dijkman B, Wertheim P, Lijmer J, van der Veen F, Bossuyt PM. The

accuracy of serum chlamydial antibodies in the diagnosis of tubal pathology: A meta-analysis. Fertility and Sterility. 1997;**67**(6):1031-1037. DOI: 10.1016/s0015-0282(97)81435-5

[14] Baseman JB, Cagle M, Korte JE, Herrera C, Rasmussen WG, Baseman JG, et al. Diagnostic assessment of Mycoplasma genitalium in culture-positive women. Journal of Clinical Microbiology. 2004;**42**(1):203-211. DOI: 10.1128/JCM.42.1.203-211.2004

[15] Vică ML, Matei HV, Siserman CV. The advantages of using multiplex PCR for the simultaneous detection of six sexually transmitted diseases. In: Samadikuchaksaraei A, editor. Polymerase Chain Reaction for Biomedical Applications. London: IntechOpen; 2016. pp. 83-100. DOI: 10.5772/65901

[16] Lee SJ, Park DC, Lee DS, Choe HS, Cho YH. Evaluation of Seeplex® STD6 ACE detection kit for the diagnosis of six bacterial sexually transmitted infections. Journal of Infection and Chemotherapy. 2012;**18**(4):494-500. DOI: 10.1007/s10156-011-0362-7

[17] Somani J, Bhullar VB, Workowski KA, Farshy CE, Black CM. Multiple drug-resistant Chlamydia trachomatis associated with clinical treatment failure. The Journal of Infectious Diseases. 2000;**181**(4):1421-1427. DOI: 10.1086/315372

[18] Mpiga P, Ravaoarinoro M. Chlamydia trachomatis persistence: An update. Microbiological Research. 2006;**161**(1):9-19. DOI: 10.1016/j.micres.2005.04.004

[19] Robertson JA, Coppola E, Heisler OR. Standardized method for determining antimicrobial susceptibility of strains of Ureaplasma urealyticum and their response to tetracycline, erythromycin, and rosaramicin. Antimicrobial Agents and Chemotherapy. 1981;**20**(1):53-58. DOI: 10.1128/AAC.20.1.53

[20] Vică ML, Matei HV, Katona A, Puia A, Teodoru CA. Molecular diagnostic of Ureaplasma urealyticum presence and tetracycline resistance in urine samples. Revista Romana de Medicina de Laborator. 2021;**29**(1):43-51. DOI: 10.2478/rrlm-2021-0006

[21] Unemo M, Shafer WM. Antimicrobial resistance in Neisseria gonorrhoeae in the 21st century: Past, evolution, and future. Clinical Microbiology Reviews. 2014;**27**(3):587-613. DOI: 10.1128/CMR.00010-14

[22] Vică ML, Glevitzky I, Glevitzky M, Siserman CV, Matei HV, Teodoru CA. Antibacterial activity of propolis extracts from the central region of romania against Neisseria gonorrhoeae. Antibiotics. 2021;**10**(6):689. DOI: 10.3390/antibiotics10060689

[23] Vică ML, Matei HV, Siserman CV. Determining the antibiotic resistance of bacterial pathogens in sexually transmitted diseases. In: Kumavath RN, editor. Antibacterial Agents. London: IntechOpen; 2017. pp. 109-127. DOI: 10.5772/67871

[24] Dubourg G, Raoult D. The challenges of preexposure prophylaxis for bacterial sexually transmitted infections. Clinical Microbiology and Infection. 2016;**22**(9):753-756. DOI: 10.1016/j.cmi.2016.08.022

[25] Russell MW, Hedges SR, Wu HY, Hook EW 3rd, Mestecky J. Mucosal immunity in the genital tract: Prospects for vaccines against sexually transmitted diseases—A review. American Journal of Reproductive Immunology. 1999;**42**(1):58-63. DOI: 10.1111/j.1600-0897.1999.tb00466.x

Chapter 2

Bacterial Sexually Transmitted Disease

Lebeza Alemu Tenaw

Abstract

Sexually transmitted diseases are among the most contagious infections caused by a variety of microorganisms such as viruses, bacteria, fungi, and protozoa. Worldwide, the incidence of bacterial sexually transmitted infections has shown a gradual increase in recent years. Common bacterial sexually transmitted diseases are Chlamydia, gonorrhea, and syphilis. Any person with signs or symptoms suggestive of bacterial sexually transmitted infections should receive a test, even if he or she does not have symptoms or know of a sex partner. Bacterial sexually transmitted diseases can be cured with the right treatment. It is important to take all medications based on the prescription to cure the sexually transmitted infection. Chlamydia is the most common bacterial sexually transmitted infection globally. Gonorrhea strains that are multi-drug resistant have been widely dispersed worldwide. Neisseria gonorrhoeae has a high level of antibiotic resistance, leading to untreatable infections that could one day pose a serious threat to public health and present the greatest obstacles to the prevention and management of sexually transmitted illnesses. Because there is no documented penicillin resistance, penicillin remains the first-line therapy for syphilis.

Keywords: sexually transmitted infections, bacterial infections, Syphilis, Chlamydia, Gonorrhea

1. Introduction

Sexually transmitted diseases (STDs), often known as "venereal diseases," are among the most contagious diseases and are caused by a variety of microorganisms that differ in symptomology, size, life cycle, and treatment susceptibility. Bacteria, viruses, fungi, and protozoa are indeed the pathogens of STDs [1, 2].

These germs can spread from one person to another through blood, sperm, vaginal, and other physiological fluids. As a result, sexually transmitted infections (STIs) are passed from one person to the next by close physical contact, primarily but not solely through sexual intercourse. Ejaculation does not have to occur for STIs to be transmitted from person to person [1, 3].

Nonsexual transmission of these infections happens often from mother to newborn during pregnancy and childbirth, through blood transfusions, and through the sharing of unsterilized needles. Any sexually active individual should discuss his or her risk factors for STIs with health professionals and ask to get a test because anyone may have an STI even without showing any symptoms [1].

Although some infections, including meningitis, can be transmitted through sexual contact, they are not considered STDs because the germs that cause meningitis can already be found in the body or in the environment, and people can get the disease for a variety of reasons [1, 2].

The prevalence of STDs remains high in poor nations, with emerging countries bearing a disproportionate share of the burden. The World Health Organization (WHO) estimates that 374 million new infections with one of four STIs will occur in 2020, which indicates that there are almost 1 million STIs acquired every day. The most prevalent STI is Chlamydia, which accounts for 129 million new infections each year. Gonorrhea has 82 million new infections per year, and syphilis has 42 million new infections annually [3].

Common bacterial STIs may affect the anorectum and perianal skin. Some of these infections are a result of the contiguous spread of sexual intercourse. Worldwide, the incidence of bacterial STIs has shown a gradual increase in recent years. The fast spread of these infections may be due to their varied clinical presentation, which includes pharyngeal, rectal, and urogenital involvement, as well as a significant number of asymptomatic cases [4, 5].

The symptoms of STIs differ between individuals depending on the causative pathogens, and commonly, many people may not experience any symptoms at all. Immediate initiation of STIs treatment is important to minimize the long-term complications of STIs and also prevent the transmission of infections to other people. Common bacterial sexually transmitted diseases are Chlamydia, gonorrhea, and syphilis [1].

2. Chlamydia

Chlamydia is a bacterial STD caused by the organism *Chlamydia trachomatis (C. trachomatis)*, an intracellular organism that produces clinical illness within 1–2 weeks after exposure, which can damage a woman's reproductive organs and cause cervicitis, urethritis, and prostatitis, which occur mostly in young (15–24-year-old) individuals, mostly prevalent in young women [6].

The infection is more likely transmitted during unprotected sexual intercourse through vaginal, anal, or oral sex with someone with the infection, even though semen does not have STI pathogens to transmit the infection from person to person. Women can get Chlamydia in the cervix, rectum, and throat. Men can get Chlamydia in the urethra, rectum, and throat [6–8]. During childbirth, chlamydial infection is also passed from mother to baby [9, 10].

For behavioral, biological, and cultural reasons, sexually active young individuals are at high risk of getting chlamydial infection. Multiple abnormalities can result from C. trachomatis infection in women including pelvic inflammatory diseases (PIDs), ectopic pregnancy, and infertility. Sometimes women receiving a diagnosis of uncomplicated cervical infection may have asymptomatic upper genital tract infection [6].

Chlamydial infection is commonly asymptomatic both in women and men. Health sector institutions frequently rely on screening tests for all sexually active women aged <25 years, and recommended annual screening for high risky individuals (women aged ≥ 25 years who have more than one sex partner, a new sex partner, or a sex partner who has an STIs) to detect chlamydial infection [2].

Chlamydia is a global public health problem that is the leading bacterial sexually transmitted infection in developed and undeveloped countries. *Nonlymphogranuloma venereum* (LGV) serovars infection is mostly asymptomatic but can produce aggressive infection manifest by perianal, anal, or rectal ulceration with resulting pain and discharge [11].

Even though evidences are insufficient to recommend routine screening for C. trachomatis among sexually active young men because of different factors (i.e., efficacy, feasibility, and cost-effectiveness), where there are clinical settings with a high prevalence of Chlamydia sexually active young men should be screened. The primary focus of women diagnosed with Chlamydia infection should be to detect and treat the infection, prevent complications, and to treat their partners, whereas men should be screened for Chlamydia only when resources permit and prevalence is high [2].

2.1 Clinical manifestation

Chlamydia trachomatis causes infection of the lower and upper genital tracts of both sexes, thus having a great influence on reproductive health. Chlamydia usually does not cause any symptoms but can still transmit the disease to others. Asymptomatic infection is frequent in women; many women with Chlamydia sampled from the cervix have no signs or symptoms of infection [6, 12].

No genital symptoms are specifically correlated with chlamydial cervical infection. But over 70% of men experience symptoms, such as urethral discharge, penile discomfort, and dysuria, which may cause serious complications that result in irreversible damage, including infertility [13].

Chlamydial infection may cause induced endocervical bleeding and mucopurulent endocervical discharge. The observation of purulent yellow or greenish cervical discharge on a cervical swab is associated with the presence of chlamydial infection [14]. When a woman does not receive treatment; Chlamydia can spread into the uterus or fallopian tubes, causing PIDs, which occur in about 10–15% of women [6, 15, 16]. In young, sexually active men, about 70% of acute epididymitis appears to be attributable to chlamydial infection [17].

2.2 Diagnosis

Since chlamydial infections may not have specific symptoms and are often indistinguishable, laboratory diagnosis is necessary to identify the correct etiology; the cell culture, and nucleic acid amplification tests (NAATs) were the gold standard tests for detection for years. Cell culture is the most sensitive test to use on easy-to-obtain specimens [10, 13].

The other most widely used diagnostic methods are the direct fluorescent antibody (DFA) and enzyme immunoassay (EIA) tests. Polymerase chain reaction (PCR) in the diagnosis of chlamydial infection has also been a gold standard [18]. Chlamydial trachomatis infection can be diagnosed by cervical or vaginal swabs or first-void urine for women, and for men can be diagnosed by testing a urethral swab or first-void urine similar to women [2].

2.3 Treatment

Chlamydia can be cured easily with antibiotic medications. Although medical treatment will cure the infection, the disease will not repair any long-term damage alone. To prevent spreading the infection to sex partners, patients starting single-dose antibiotic therapy should not have sex until the treatment is completed [6]. In some cases, chlamydial infection recurs 3–6 weeks after treatment [19].

- Adolescent and adult chlamydial infection treatment regimen: doxycycline 100 mg orally two times/day for 7 days; alternatively; azithromycin 1 g orally in a single-dose or levofloxacin 500 mg orally once daily for 7 days are recommended.

- Azithromycin 1 g orally in a single dose is recommended for chlamydial infection during pregnancy or amoxicillin 500 mg orally three times per day for 7 days.

- The following is the recommended treatment regimen for neonatal chlamydial infection: Erythromycin base or ethyl succinate 50 mg/kg body weight per day, divided into four doses per day for 14 days

- For pregnant women with chlamydial infection, a single dose of azithromycin 1 g orally is recommended, and alternatively amoxicillin 500 mg orally three times a day for 7 days [2].

3. Additional management considerations

An individual treated for Chlamydia infection should be instructed to abstain from sexual intercourse for 7 days after single-dose therapy to minimize disease transmission to their sexual partners. To minimize the risk of reinfection, an infected person should abstain from sexual intercourse until all of their sex partners have been treated.

Multiple coinfections may happen when a person receives a diagnosis of Chlamydia infection and should be tested for human immunodeficiency virus *(HIV),* syphilis, and gonorrhea. Test of cure to detect therapeutic failure is not advised for non-pregnant persons treated with the recommended unless therapeutic adherence is in question, reinfection is suspected or symptoms persist. If an individual had sexual contact with chlamydial infected person, the sex partners of the infected person should be referred for evaluation, testing, and presumptive treatment [2].

4. Gonorrhea

Gonorrhea is an STD that is caused by the bacterium *Neisseria Gonorrhoeae* (*N. gonorrhoeae*) that can infect all individuals. Gram-negative diplococcus, *N. gonorrhoeae,* is initially identified in 1879 by Albert Neisser from exudates of urethritis and cervicitis. Humans are the only natural reservoir of *N. gonorrhoeae* with an incubation period of 1–14 days [5, 20].

It can cause infections in the genitals, rectum, and throat, which affect young people ages 15–24 years. Men who experience symptomatic urethral infections may seek curative therapy, whereas women frequently experience asymptomatic infections caused by *N. gonorrhoeae*. Asymptomatic infection from *N. Gonorrhoeae* may affect the women's urethra, endocervix, rectum, and pharynx, which make up the main reservoir for gonococcal infection [21].

Gonorrhea can spread by having sexual contact with an infected person, and from mother to child during childbirth. Gonorrhea is the second commonly reported bacterial sexually transmitted diseases, and the incidence of new cases of gonorrhea is especially high in developing countries, which can produce symptoms in men that cause them to seek curative treatment to prevent complications [22, 23].

Annual screening for *N. Gonorrhoeae* infection is recommended for all sexually active women aged <25 years and for older women at increased risk for infection. Risk factors for gonorrheal infection include inconsistent condom use among persons who are not in mutually monogamous relationships, exchanging sex for money, and coexisting STIs [2].

4.1 Clinical manifestation

Gonorrhea may have no symptoms, but some men may have a burning sensation when urinating; white, yellow, or green discharge from the penis; painful or swollen testicles, and some women may often have a painful or burning sensation when urinating; increased vaginal discharge/vaginal bleeding, which may have a risk of developing serious complications [24].

If gonorrhea is not appropriately treated, it can lead to pelvic inflammatory disease, infertility, and ectopic pregnancy. Pregnant women can pass the gonorrheal infection to their babies during childbirth, and the newborn can become blind or have life-threatening infections as a result [21].

Anorectal gonococcal infection shows a thick purulent discharge that is expressed from the anal crypts in response to external anal pressure. Nonspecific findings of mucosal erythema, edema, friability, and pus are noted in infected individuals with proctitis from rectal infection [4].

4.2 Diagnosis

Specific microbiologic diagnosis of *N. gonorrhoeae* infection should be performed for all persons at risk of having gonorrhea, which can potentially reduce many related complications [2]. Urine can be used to test for ureteral infection of gonorrhea. However, if there is oral and/or anal sex, swabs may be used to collect samples from the throat, rectum, and cervix. Cell culture, nucleic acid hybridization tests (NAHTs), and nucleic acid amplification tests (NAATs) are available for the detection of genitourinary infection with *N. gonorrhoeae* [20].

The standard diagnostic procedure for men with symptomatic urethritis is the gram stain, because of its high specificity and sensitivity. However, in asymptomatic men or women with genital infections, the Gram stain is less useful because of its lower sensitivity. Gram stain of endocervical specimens, pharyngeal specimens, or rectal specimens is not sufficient to detect infection and therefore is not recommended [25].

The result of cultural diagnosis may be reduced if lubricants with antibacterial agents are used during anoscopy, which makes water a recommended lubricant in this setting. There are no approved nucleic acid amplification tests for rectal infection, while nonculture techniques are gaining acceptance in genital gonococcal infections [26].

Certain NAATs that have been demonstrated to detect Neisseria species might have low specificity when diagnosing oropharyngeal specimens for *N. Gonorrhoeae* but

NAAT sensitivity for identifying *N. Gonorrhoeae* from nongenital and urogenital sites is superior to culture even though it may vary by NAAT type. Optimal specimen types for gonorrhea screening using NAATs include vaginal swab specimens for women and first-void urine for men [27].

4.3 Treatment

Gonorrhea treatment is complicated by the ability of *N. Gonorrhoeae* to develop resistance to antimicrobials. There is a high level of antimicrobial resistance in *N. Gonorrhoeae,* resulting in untreatable infections that in the future may become a significant major public health issue and pose the greatest challenges to the prevention and control of sexually transmitted infections [20].

Many of the previously recommended therapies are no longer effective, which makes treatment opportunities for *N. Gonorrhoeae* limited. Therefore, new dual antimicrobial treatment regimens are urgently needed [20, 28]. Zoliflodacin is the new recommended oral antibiotic that successfully treats most cases of uncomplicated gonorrhea [21].

- Recommendation regimen for gonorrheal infection of the pharynx, cervix, urethra, or rectum that is not complicated. If chlamydial infection has not been ruled out, treat for 7 days with doxycycline 100 mg orally twice a day.

- Alternative regimens if ceftriaxone is not available; gentamicin 240 mg IM in a single-dose, plus azithromycin 2 g orally in a single dose, or cefixime 800 mg orally in a single-dose [2].

5. Antimicrobial-resistant *N. gonorrhoeae*

Gonorrhea treatment may be complicated by the ability of *N. gonorrhoeae* specious to develop resistance to antimicrobials drugs. Due to the emerging antimicrobial resistance dual therapy for gonorrhea with a cephalosporin plus either azithromycin or doxycycline, even if NAAT for C. trachomatis was negative at the time of treatment recommended by the center for disease control in 2010. Azithromycin might predispose to resistance due to its prolonged half-life [27].

6. Syphilis

Syphilis is one of the most prevalent bacterial STDs caused by the *Treponema pallidum T. pallidum) bacterium*. It infects the genital area, lips, mouth, or anus of both men and women. Syphilis is transmitted between people by direct contact with a syphilis sore during vaginal, anal, or oral sex and can spread from a mother with syphilis to her unborn baby during pregnancy and childbirth. It is not transmitted through the use of the same toilet; wearing the patient's clothes, or even using food utensils [12].

It is a contagious disease that can cause serious health problems, such as arthritis, brain damage, dementia, and blindness, and may lead to death if left untreated. Syphilis is often difficult to diagnose, and the patient may not have any symptoms for years [1].

T. pallidum can infect the central nervous system at any stage of syphilis that result in neurosyphilis. Early neurologic clinical manifestations of syphilitic meningitis are usually present within the first few months of infection. Late neurologic manifestations occur 10 to >30 years after infection. Ocular syphilis and otosyphilis can occur at any stage of syphilis but are commonly identified during the early stages and can occur with or without central nervous system (CNS) involvement [2].

6.1 Stages of Syphilis

Syphilis infection is divided into four stages with different symptoms that appear in the patient. The symptoms and signs associated with each stage may overlap each other, and symptoms may not appear in order. Some patients have not had any symptoms for years. After the initial infection, the bacterium *T. pallidum* can remain inactive in the body before becoming active many times, and it needs 21 days to show the first symptom after the acquisition of a syphilis infection [5, 29].

Primary syphilis: During the primary stage of syphilis, a single sore or multiple sores may be noticed, which usually lasts 3–6 weeks and heals regardless of taking the treatment. The primary stage of anorectal syphilis that comes through anal intercourse appears within 2–10 weeks of exposure. The anal chancre is a small indurated papule that eventually upgraded to anal ulcers; located on the perianal skin or in the anal canal; may be single or multiple; are associated with painless but prominent inguinal lymphadenopathy but heals without treatment in 2–4 weeks. Anal ulcers contrasts with genital ulcers are frequently painful [30, 31]. Even after the sore goes away, continuing the treatment is recommended; this will stop the infection from moving to the secondary stage [29].

Secondary syphilis: Four to ten weeks after primary syphilis appears, the spreading of hematogenous untreated syphilis infection leads to secondary stage syphilis [4]. During the secondary stage, the patient may have skin rashes and/or mucous membrane lesions. The rash can appear 2–8 weeks after the chancre develops and sometimes before it heals. The rash may look like rough, red, or reddish-brown spots on the bottoms of the feet and the palms of the hands. This rash does not usually cause itching, but it may be accompanied by wart-like sores in the mouth and sexual areas [29].

The infection is highly contagious during this stage. The symptoms at this stage will go away when the treatment is initiated. Without the right treatment, the infection will move to the latent and tertiary stages of syphilis [1, 5, 29]. The majority of untreated symptoms of syphilis spontaneously resolve after 12 weeks. One-fourth of these untreated patients will experience early latent syphilis [4].

Latent syphilis: The latent stage of syphilis is a period when there are no visible signs or symptoms. Without treatment, the infected person continues to have syphilis in his/her body for years. The infection is contagious in the early part of the latent stage and may continue its transmission even without showing symptoms [1, 29].

Tertiary/Late syphilis: This is the most destructive stage, in which complications of syphilis appear in patients who have not undergone the required treatment. Tertiary syphilis is very serious and would occur 10–30 years after the infection began. In tertiary syphilis, the disease damages the internal organs, which results in death [1, 4, 29].

6.2 Diagnosis

Dark field microscopic examinations and molecular tests for detecting *T. Pallidum* directly from lesion exudate are methods for diagnosing early syphilis and congenital syphilis. Another method for diagnosis is the demonstration of spirochetes in biopsy specimens stained with Warthin-Starry Silver. Alternatively, a direct fluorescent antibody test for *T. Pallidum* is performed by some laboratories (11,25).

A nontreponemal test (i.e., venereal disease research laboratory [VDRL] or rapid plasma reagin [RPR] test) and a treponemal test (*Treponema pallidum* passive particle agglutination [TP-PA] assay), chemiluminescence immunoassays [CIAs] and immunoblots, or rapid treponemal assays are the diagnostic methods of syphilis [4, 29].

6.3 Treatment

- For adults and adolescents with primary, secondary, or early latent syphilis; benzathine penicillin (G 2.4 million units) is administered intramuscularly in a single dose.

- For adults and adolescents with late latent syphilis or latent syphilis of unknown duration; benzathine penicillin G 7.2 million units total, administered as three doses of 2.4 million units each administered intramuscularly at weekly intervals.

- For neurosyphilis, ocular syphilis, or otosyphilis; aqueous crystalline penicillin G 18–24 million units per day, administered as 3–4 million units intravenously every 4 hours or continuous infusion for 10–14 days [2, 32].

7. Additional management options

All individuals who have primary and secondary syphilis are encouraged to take an HIV test at the time of diagnosis and treatment and recommended to offered HIV PrEP for negative HIV test results. Persons who have symptomatic neurologic syphilis disease should have an evaluation that includes cerebral spinal fluid analysis and individuals with syphilis who have symptoms of ocular syphilis should have cranial nerve and ophthalmologic examinations [2].

8. Follow-Up

Clinical and serologic investigations should be needed within 12 months of treatment; if conditions for follow-up are uncertain more frequent evaluation might be prudent. Assessing serologic response to treatment can be difficult, and definitive criteria for evaluating treatment outcomes by serologic criteria have not been well established [33].

In addition, nontreponemal test titers might decrease more slowly for persons previously treated for syphilis. Among individuals with neurologic findings without any reported sexual exposure during the previous 3–6 months indicating that treatment failure might be possible, a cerebral spinal fluid examination is recommended, and should also be reevaluated for HIV infection [34].

9. Prevention of bacterial STDs

Abstain: When there is no open discussion about a sexual partner's past sexual health history, abstaining from sexual activity is the most efficient strategy to avoid STIs.

Communicate and double-check: Always discuss safe sex prior participating in just about any substantial sexual contact. Because sexually transmitted illnesses do not often show symptoms, it is possible to be infected without realizing it. So, avoid vaginal and anal intercourse before checking for STDs. Oral sex was not without risks, but it is less dangerous. To avoid direct touch, use a latex condom or a dental dam.

Use condoms and dental dams consistently: If abstinence is not the first choice, use latex condoms to decrease the possibility of getting infected with sexually transmitted illnesses. When using a latex condom or dental dam, avoid using petroleum lubricants like petroleum jelly. Furthermore, condoms composed of natural membranes are ineffective at preventing STDs.

Avoid excessive alcohol or drugs: People who are prone to consuming excessive alcohol or drugs are more likely to take sexual risks [5].

Conflict of interest

The authors declare no conflict of interest.

Abbreviations

CNS	Central Nervous System
CIAs	Chemiluminescence Immunoassays
DFA	Direct Fluorescent Antibody
EIA	Enzyme Immunoassay
LGV	Nonlymphogranuloma Venereum
NAATs	Nucleic acid amplification tests
RPR	Rapid Plasma Regain
STDs	Sexually Transmitted Diseases
STIs	Sexually Transmitted Infections
TP-PA	*Treponema* Pallidum Passive Particle Agglutination
VDRL	Venereal Disease Research Laboratory
WHO	World Health Organization

Author details

Lebeza Alemu Tenaw
Department of Reproductive Health, College of Health Sciences, Woldia University, Woldia, Ethiopia

*Address all correspondence to: lebezaa@gmail.com

References

[1] National Institutes of Health (NIH). Sexually Transmitted Diseases (STDs). 2015. Available from: https://www.nichd.nih.gov/health/topics/factsheets/stds

[2] Workowski KA et al. Sexually transmitted infections treatment guidelines. MMWR - Recommendations and Reports. 2021;**70**(4):1

[3] World Health Organization(WHO). Fact Sheets of Sexually transmitted infections (STIs). 2021. Available from: https://www.who.int/news-room/fact-sheets/detail/sexually-transmitted-infections-(stis)

[4] Whitlow CB. Bacterial sexually transmitted diseases. Clinics in Colon and Rectal Surgery. 2004;**17**(04):209-214

[5] Buder S et al. Bacterial sexually transmitted infections. JDDG: Journal der Deutschen Dermatologischen Gesellschaft. 2019;**17**(3):287-315

[6] Centers for Disease Control and Prevention(CDC). Sexually transmited disease: Chlamydia - fact sheet. 2022

[7] Sorvillo FJ, Lieb LE, Waterman SH. Incidence of campylobacteriosis among patients with AIDS in Los Angeles County. Journal of Acquired Immune Deficiency Syndromes. 1991;**4**(6):598-602

[8] STAMM WE et al. Chlamydia trachomatis urethral infections in men: Prevalence, risk factors, and clinical manifestations. Annals of Internal Medicine. 1984;**100**(1):47-51

[9] Rompalo AM. Diagnosis and treatment of sexually acquired proctitis and proctocolitis: An update. Clinical Infectious Diseases. 1999;**28**(1):S84-S90

[10] Brunham RC et al. The unexpected impact of a Chlamydia trachomatis infection control program on susceptibility to reinfection. The Journal of Infectious Diseases. 2005;**192**(10):1836-1844

[11] Meštrović T, Ljubin-Sternak S. Molecular mechanisms of Chlamydia trachomatis resistance to antimicrobial drugs. Frontiers in Bioscience. 2018;**23**:656-670

[12] Medicine Plus. Chlamydia. National Liberary of Medicine; 2016

[13] Ljubin-Sternak S, Meštrović T. Chlamydia trachomatis and genital mycoplasmas: Pathogens with an impact on human reproductive health. Journal of Pathogens. 2014;**2014**

[14] Brunham RC et al. Mucopurulent cervicitis—the ignored counterpart in women of urethritis in men. New England Journal of Medicine. 1984;**311**(1):1-6

[15] Orle KA et al. Simultaneous PCR detection of Haemophilus ducreyi, Treponema pallidum, and herpes simplex virus types 1 and 2 from genital ulcers. Journal of Clinical Microbiology. 1996;**34**(1):49-54

[16] Handsfield HH et al. Differences in the therapeutic response of chlamydia-positive and chlamydia-negative forms of nongonococcal urethritis. Journal of the American Venereal Disease Association. 1976:5-9

[17] Oriel J et al. Infection with chlamydia group A in men with urethritis due to Neisseria gonorrhoeae. Journal of Infectious Diseases. 1975;**131**(4):376-382

[18] Black CM. Current methods of laboratory diagnosis of Chlamydia trachomatis infections. Clinical Microbiology Reviews. 1997;**10**(1):160-184

[19] Ossewaarde J et al. Efficacy of single-dose azithromycin versus doxycycline in the treatment of cervical infections caused byChlamydia trachomatis. European Journal of Clinical Microbiology and Infectious Diseases. 1992;**11**(8):693-697

[20] Workowski KA. Centers for Disease Control and Prevention sexually transmitted diseases treatment guidelines. Clinical Infectious Diseases. 2015;**61**(8):S759-S762

[21] National Institutes of Health(NIH). Novel Antibiotic Shows Promise in Treatment of Uncomplicated Gonorrhea. 2018

[22] Kampmeier RH. Identification of the gonococcus by Albert Neisser. Sexually Transmitted Diseases. 1978;**5**(2):71-72

[23] Kampmeier R. Introduction of sulfonamide therapy for gonorrhea. Sexually Transmitted Diseases. 1983;**10**(2):81-84

[24] Holmes KK, Johnson DW, Trostle HJ. An estimate of the risk of men acquiring gonorrhea by sexual contact with infected females. American Journal of Epidemiology. 1970;**91**(2):170-174

[25] Johnson RE et al. Screening tests to detect Chlamydia trachomatis and Neisseria gonorrhoeae infections. MMWR Recommended Reports. 2002;**51**(15):1-38

[26] Young H, Manavi K, McMillan A. Evaluation of ligase chain reaction for the non-cultural detection of rectal and pharyngeal gonorrhoea in men who have sex with men. Sexually Transmitted Infections. 2003 Dec;**79**(6):484-486. DOI: 10.1136/sti.79.6.484. PMID: 14663126; PMCID: PMC1744765

[27] Papp JR, Schachter J, Gaydos CA, Van Der Pol B. Recommendations for the laboratory-based detection of Chlamydia trachomatis and Neisseria gonorrhoeae—2014. MMWR. Recommendations and reports: Morbidity and mortality weekly report. Recommendations and Reports/Centers for Disease Control. 2014 Mar 3;**63**:1

[28] Queirós CS, da Costa JB. Gonorrhea: Antimicrobial resistance and new drugs. Journal of the Portuguese Society of Dermatology and Venereology. 2019;**77**(3):233-238

[29] Centers for Disease Control and Prevention(CDC). Sexually Transmited Disease: Syphilis-Fact Sheet. 2022

[30] Crosby RA, Charnigo RA, Weathers C, Caliendo AM, Shrier LA. Condom effectiveness against non-viral sexually transmitted infections: a prospective study using electronic daily diaries. Sexually Transmitted Infections. 2012 Nov 1;**88**(7):484-489

[31] Winer RL, Hughes JP, Feng Q, O'Reilly S, Kiviat NB, Holmes KK, Koutsky LA. Condom use and the risk of genital human papillomavirus infection in young women. New England Journal of Medicine. 2006 Jun 22;**354**(25):2645-2654

[32] Kohl KS et al. Usefulness of partner notification for syphilis control. Sexually Transmitted Diseases. 1999:201-207

[33] Ghanem KG, Erbelding EJ, Wiener ZS, Rompalo AM. Serological response to syphilis treatment in HIV-positive and HIV-negative patients attending sexually transmitted diseases clinics. Sexually Transmitted Infections. 2007 Apr 1;**83**(2):97-101

[34] Sena AC, Wolff M, Martin DH, Behets F, Van Damme K, Leone P, et al. Predictors of serological cure and serofast state after treatment in HIV-negative persons with early syphilis. Clinical Infectious Diseases. 2011 Dec 1;**53**(11):1092-1099

Chapter 3

Sexually Transmitted Diseases in Pediatrics

Diana Leticia Coronel Martínez and Luis Augusto Moya Barquín

Abstract

The scope of this chapter would be describing bacterial sexually transmitted diseases that are of interest in pediatric population such as gonorrhea and syphilis. Currently, this diseases has been reported an increased incidence mostly in adolescents in different regions around the world such as Australia and United States. These diseases sometimes considered anecdotal are always difficult to manage because they are considered taboos; diagnosis and treatment are challenging because of the interaction with the child and his/her parents. Other diseases such as chlamydia are also taking a great importance in populations from 10 to 24 years old due to the high transmission, high incidence, and complications such as infertility, almost 80% or chlamydia infections are asymptomatic in women being one of the leading causes of infertility that could be permanent. In this chapter, we will be discussing about the main factors of this diseases, how to manage from pediatric perspective, the most novel diagnostic tests and treatments (if available), and any vaccine development possibilities.

Keywords: syphilis, gonorrhea, chlamydia, trichomoniasis, sexually transmitted diseases, sexual abuse

1. Introduction

Sexually transmitted diseases (STDs) surveillance is key to understand the surveillance and the burden of these diseases in pediatrics. In this chapter, we will be presenting the key features of bacterial sexually transmitted diseases in general and focus on the pediatric population. Pediatric aspects of sexually transmitted diseases are important because these are the basis for the development of new public health tools for prevention. Most of these diseases can be treated; nevertheless, the continuous use of antibiotic therapy is already giving trouble with antibiotic resistance as it is the case of gonorrhea. New generations have a more open sexual behavior and are also starting earlier sexual contacts, which makes crucial the development of new ways of sexual education and the development of vaccines that can be started in younger populations.

2. Epidemiology

In 2016, the World Health Organization (WHO) estimated the global prevalence and incidence of bacterial sexually transmitted diseases in population from 15 to 49 years of age; for this estimation, almost 130 studies were reviewed. The estimated prevalence for Chlamydia, Trichomonas, Syphilis, and Gonorrhea taking into account the prevalence data from 2009 to 2016 and per gender is presented in **Table 1**. The prevalence of these diseases is inversely proportional to the income in the countries and regions; with higher incomes, the prevalence goes lower. Incidence of these pathogens per gender is presented in **Table 2** [1].

In the 2020 National Surveillance of STDs in the United States, a total of 1,579,885 cases of Chlamydia trachomatis infection were reported to the CDC, making it the most common notifiable sexually transmitted infection in the United States for that year. This case count corresponds to a rate of 481.3 per 100,000 population; for syphilis, 133,945 cases were reported including 41,655 cases of primary and secondary syphilis, the most infectious stages of the disease. Since 2000, rates of primary and secondary syphilis have increased among men, likely attributable to increases in cases among men having sex with men (MSM). For Gonorrhea, a total of 677,769 cases were reported do the CDC, making it the second most common notifiable sexually transmitted infection in the United States for that year. In the case of Trichomoniasis, in 2018, 2.6 million infections were reported; this pathogen can increase the risk of HIV and preterm deliveries with low birth weight. The prevalence of Trichomonas vaginalis in the United States is 2.1% among women aged 14–59 and 0.5% among men (representative sample from 2013 to2016). If we compare 2016 report with the 2020 report, it seems that there was a decrease in the number of cases; but this is indeed an artifact due to COVID-19 pandemic. Even in the face of COVID-19, an important number of STDs were reported; [2, 3] number of cases by selected groups of age and from this survey (Trichomoniasis was not included) are presented in **Table 3**.

From **Table 3**, Chlamydia, Gonorrhea, and Syphilis cases start rising at 15 years of age; with the highest peak from 20 to 24 years of age; 25–29 years, it is still higher, and the cases start to decline at 30 years of age and keep decreasing. This epidemiological

Gender	WHO 2016 estimated global prevalence, % (95% UI-uncertainty index)			
	Chlamydia	Gonorrhea	Trichomoniasis	Syphilis
Women	3.8 (3.3–4.5)	0.9 (0.7–1.1)	5.3 (4.0–7.2)	0.5 (0.5–0.6)
Men	2.7 (1.9–3.7)	0.7 (0.5–1.1)	0.6 (0.4–0.9)	0.5 (0.4–0.6)

Table 1.
2016 WHO prevalence estimates of chlamydia, gonorrhea, Trichomoniasis, and syphilis, global by gender.

Gender	WHO 2016 estimated global incidence, cases per 1000 (95% UI-uncertainty index)			
	Chlamydia	Gonorrhea	Trichomoniasis	Syphilis
Women	34 (25–45)	20 (14–28)	40 (27–58)	1.7 (1.4–2.0)
Men	33 (21–48)	26 (15–41)	42 (23–69)	1.6 (1.3–1.9)

Table 2.
2016 WHO incidence estimates of chlamydia, gonorrhea, Trichomoniasis, and syphilis, global by gender.

Age group (years)	Rates per 100,000 of reported cases by age group, gender, and disease United States, 2020					
	Chlamydia		Gonorrhea		Syphilis	
	Male	Female	Male	Female	Male	Female
10–14	11.3	85.4	5.5	23.3	0.1	0.2
15–19	846.3	2857.9	369.0	616.4	10.9	5.9
20–24	1627.3	3729.6	821.5	866.9	43.5	14.3
25–29	988.3	1548.0	727.9	505.3	58.1	14.4
30–34	611.7	713.3	567.6	312.3	55.7	13.0
35–39	340.7	332.3	357.4	180.6	39.4	9.1
40–44	203.3	168.5	240.3	101.5	29.9	7.3
45–54	98.8	59.7	124.7	37.0	21.0	3.4
55–64	38.7	16.5	57.0	9.4	11.4	0.9
65+	6.4	2.0	10.3	1.1	2.1	0.1
Total	339.4	616.5	238.5	174.5	20.8	4.7

Table 3.
Sexually transmitted disease CDC surveillance 2020 (adapted from the CDC report, division of STD prevention).

behavior is the basis of the development of public health measurements, treatment, and eventually, vaccine development.

3. The pathogens

Bacteria causing STDs have similar features related to their biology and mechanisms of infection. C. trachomatis (CT) is a Gram-negative obligate intracellular bacterium discovered in 1907, humans are its exclusive natural host; serovars associated with sexually transmitted infection are D–K. Chlamydiae are obligate intracellular bacteria with two development forms, the infectious elementary body (EB) and the active division body that is not infectious, reticulate body (RB). Once a cell is infected, the EBs can differentiate to RBs, and after a cycle of around 2 days, more EBs can be released by lysis of the host cell or by the active release of inclusions [4–7]. Neisseria gonorrhea (Ng) is also a Gram-negative bacterium obligated human pathogen described for the first time by Albert Neisser on 1879. CDC provides data on reported gonorrhea morbidity since the 1940s. Ng has evolved mechanisms for evading innate immunity and suppressing adaptive immune responses, like CT [8–10].

Syphilis pathogen is a spirochaete, Treponema pallidum (Tp); analysis based on the mutation rates of this pathogen suggests that venereal syphilis diverged several thousand years ago from Africa; this contradicts the Columbian hypothesis, in which the idea was that the shipmates of Christopher Columbus "Cristóbal Colón" brought the newly evolved venereal disease from the New World into Western Europe in the late fifteenth century; again like CT and Ng, Tp is an obligate human pathogen [11, 12].

Even the title of this chapter refers to bacterial STDs, Trichomonas vaginalis (Tv) deserved to be included since it is the most prevalent curable STD globally. Tv is a flagellated protozoan parasite of the human genital tract. Tv has no cystic stage in its life cycle, four anterior flagella provide the parasite its characteristic motility, and its single posterior flagellum assists the motility of extracellular nutrients toward the cytosome of the cell [13].

4. The disease

4.1 Pathogenesis and transmission

All the included pathogens are highly transmissible, one of the most important features for this is that most of the infected people, mostly women, remain asymptomatic and do not seek treatment. All of these diseases are transmitted during sexual intercourse.

CT can avoid destruction by the host's innate and adaptive immune systems by autophagy, which allows CT to migrate to the upper genital tract for establishing a chronic infection. Without treatment, up to 50% of infected women will continue to be infected for greater than 1 year. CT can be in the semen of infected males or can be released from infected female genital tract epithelial cell. CT can bind to almost all receptors in the epithelial cell (i.e. mannose, mannose-6-phosphate, epidermal growth factor, B1 integrin, platelet-derived growth factor receptor, protein disulfide isomerase, fibroblast growth factor receptor, and ephrin receptor A2). CT induces actin remodeling that facilitates the entry in the cytoplasm. The EBs are internalized in vacuoles and form an intracytoplasmic inclusion, which can evolve to RBs, these RBs are the non-infectious replicative form and use nutrients within the host cytoplasm and replicate by binary fission, when the RB-filled inclusion reaches critical volume, RBs convert back to EBs, and they can be released to the extracellular milieu by two mechanisms: host lysis or extrusion of the cytoplasmic inclusion [4, 14].

Ng affects the urogenital tract, mostly the columnar and transitional epithelia. Ng prevents complement activation, opsonization, and bacterial killing. Ng prevents complement activation, opsonization, and bacterial killing and can survive in and around the macrophages and neutrophils during infection and modulate the immune-activating properties of dendritic cells. Ng infection does not generate immunological memory, owing to the ability of Ng antigenically and phase vary its surface structures. In men, Ng attaches to sperm, which is easily transmitted from men to their partners through ejaculates with high number of bacteria. In women, bacterial sialidases, which are secreted by the cervicovaginal microbiota of women, must first desialylate Ng lipooligosaccharide to enable efficient transmission [10].

In the case of Tp, the mechanisms of tissue damage by Tp are still not well described. The local inflammation process has been attributed to the spirochete itself; nevertheless, the fragility and low protein content of its outer membrane make it very difficult to well characterize them. A well definition of protective immunity is still unavailable. Transmission of venereal syphilis occurs during sexual contact with an actively infected partner, same as the other three diseases described in this chapter; with only 10 organisms in the exudate, the disease can be transmitted. Tp can penetrate directly the mucous membranes and adhere to the epithelial cells and extracellular matrix components for establishing the infection, fibronectin and laminin are key for Tp interactions with the cell. The infection becomes systemic very fast, once the blood–brain barrier is reached (this happens in as many as 40% of individuals with syphilis), early syphilis without treatment can cause severe neurological complications [12].

Tv transmission occurs almost exclusively via sexual contact, even some transmission via fomites has been argued, which is highly controversial and lacks strong evidence. During sexual intercourse, Tv in the genital tract of the infected partner is transferred to the uninfected partner, when Tv reaches the epithelial cells, Tv assumes an ameboid form increasing its surface area contact. The five primary surface adhesins responsible for the attachment of the parasite to the epithelia are AP120, AP65, AP51, AP33, and AP23. Iron is the most important mediator of Tv growth [13].

4.2 Clinical manifestations

It can be said that all these diseases have similar clinical manifestations including purulent exudates in male urethra and female cervix and urinary tract infection manifestations. Also, one common feature is that all of them can be asymptomatic, at least for some time. Common clinical manifestations are presented in **Table 4** for comparison purposes. Special characteristics are described in the next subsections.

4.2.1 Chlamydia in pediatrics

4.2.1.1 Chlamydia neonatorum

Chlamydia can be presented in different age groups in pediatrics. In the neonate, it is also known as Chlamydia neonatorum. Infection in neonates results from perinatal exposure to the mother's infected cervix. Initial infection involves the mucous membranes of the eye, oropharynx, urogenital tract, and rectum, although infection might be asymptomatic in these locations. The most common manifestation in neonates is conjunctivitis that develops 5–12 days after birth. Nowadays, this infection is much less frequent due to widespread prenatal screening and treatment of pregnant women.

4.2.1.2 Chlamydial pneumonia among infants

This type of pneumonia typically occurs at age 1–3 months and is a subacute pneumonia. Characteristic signs include a repetitive staccato cough with tachypnea and hyperinflation and bilateral diffuse infiltrates on a chest radiograph. Peripheral eosinophilia ($\geq$400 cells/mm3) occurs frequently. Considering that this clinical presentation is broad, symptoms of pneumonia in infants aged 1–3 months and especially those whose mothers have a history of are at risk for or suspected of having a chlamydial infection should be tested for C. trachomatis and treated if infected. Mothers at risk include aged $<$25 years and those aged $\geq$25 years who have a new sex partner, more than one sex partner, a sex partner with concurrent partners, or a sex partner who has or had a sexually transmitted disease/infection.

4.2.2 Neisseria gonorrhea in pediatrics

4.2.2.1 Neisseria gonorrhea in neonates

In the neonatal period, infections due to Ng result from perinatal exposure to the infected cervix of the mother.

Ophthalmia neonatorum can result in perforation of the globe of the eye and blindness. Newborns at increased risk for gonococcal ophthalmia include those who did not receive ophthalmic prophylaxis and whose mothers had no prenatal care, have

Clinical manifestation	CT	Ng	Tp	Tv
Can be asymptomatic?	Yes, very frequent mainly in females	Yes, very frequent mainly in females	Varied and often subtle manifestations, it is called the Great Imitator. First manifestation could be a single ulcer (chancre) or multiple lesions typically painless with regional lymphadenopathy ~3 weeks post-infection that resolves spontaneously	Yes in 50% of the cases and around 30% of them can develop some symptoms in the 6-month period postinfection
Itching, pain during intercourse, frothy discharge, vaginitis in women, mild to severe and urethritis with purulent discharge in men; urinary tract infection symptoms in both	Yes	Yes	No	Yes, In acute cases, punctate hemorrhagic spots may be present on the vaginal and cervical mucosa (colpitis macularis, or "strawberry cervix")
Pelvic inflammatory disease	Yes	Yes	No	Yes
Cervical cancer association	No	No	No	Yes
Infertility	Yes	Yes	Yes	Yes
Vertical transmission?	Yes	Yes	Yes	Yes
Extragenital infections are present	Yes (pharyngitis and proctitis)	Yes (pharyngitis and proctitis)	Ocular syphilis and Otosyphilis can occur at any stage but is commonly identified during the early stages and can present with or without additional Central Nervous System involvement	
Other special features	Co-infection with Ng is frequent	Co-infection with CT is frequent	Ocular syphilis can result in permanent vision loss. Otosyphilis typically presents with cochleo-vestibular symptoms, including tinnitus, vertigo, and sensorineural hearing loss. Hearing loss can be unilateral or bilateral, have a sudden onset, progress rapidly, and can result in permanent hearing loss	

Table 4.
Common clinical features of sexually transmitted diseases (CT, ng, Tp, and Tv).

a history sexually transmitted infections or history of substance abuse. A Gram stain of the conjunctival exudate will be very helpful for a strong suspicion under the finding of intracellular Gram-negative diplococci. This finding can justify the treatment for gonorrhea, appropriate cultures and antimicrobial susceptibility testing for Neisseria gonorrhoeae will be required.

Neonates can develop disseminated gonococcal infection that can be presented as sepsis, arthritis, or meningitis. It is a rare complication of neonatal gonococcal infection. Localized gonococcal infection of the scalp can result from fetal monitoring through scalp electrodes. Detecting gonococcal infection when suspected in neonates will require cultures of blood, cerebrospinal fluid, or joint aspirate. Positive Gram-stained smears of different specimens are considered strong evidence for initiating treatment for Ng.

Another important consideration is neonates born to mothers with untreated gonorrhea. These neonates should be tested and treated for Ng.

4.2.3 Syphilis

Special considerations for Syphilis must be taken considering the different clinical stages at presentation. Primary syphilis classically presents as a single painless ulcer or chancre at the site of infection but can also present with multiple, atypical, or painful lesions. Secondary syphilis manifestations can include skin rash, mucocutaneous lesions, and lymphadenopathy. Tertiary syphilis can present with cardiac involvement, gummatous lesions, tabes dorsalis, and general paresis. Latent infections are those lacking clinical manifestations and are detected by serologic testing; if this was acquired within the preceding year it is referred to as early latent syphilis; all other cases of latent syphilis are classified as late latent syphilis or latent syphilis of unknown duration [2–16].

4.2.3.1 Syphilis in pediatrics

Infants and children aged ≥1 month with diagnosis of syphilis required to be evaluated for determine if syphilis is congenital or acquired, when primary or secondary syphilis is determined, children need to be evaluated by an interdisciplinary group including a general pediatrician, an pediatric infectious disease specialist, psychologist, social workers, and other specialists depending on the required treatment. Sexual abuse must be investigated.

In the case of latent syphilis, cerebrospinal fluid must be evaluated in addition to the considerations done for primary and secondary.

4.2.3.1.1 Congenital syphilis

Maternal risk factors for syphilis during pregnancy include sex with multiple partners, sex in conjunction with drug use or transactional sex, late entry to prenatal care or no prenatal care, methamphetamine or heroine use, incarceration of the woman or her partner, and unstable housing or homelessness.

All neonates born to mothers who have reactive non-treponemal and treponemal test results should be evaluated with quantitative non-treponemal serologic test performed on the neonate's serum (umbilical cord blood has to be avoided due to the presence of maternal blood), and Wharton's jelly could lead to a false-negative result.

Congenital Syphilis	Physical examination	Serum non-treponemal serologic test	Dark field test or PCR of placenta, cord, lesions, or body fluids	Silver stain of the placenta or cord	Recommended evaluation
Proven or highly probable	Abnormal and consistent with congenital syphilis	Fourfold or greater, higher than the mother's titer at delivery	Positive	Positive	Cerebrospinal fluid (CSF) analysis for VDRL, cell count and protein. Complete blood count (CBC) and differential and platelet count. Long-bone radiographs
Possible	Normal	Equal to or less than fourfold of the maternal titer at delivery*	NA	NA	
Less Likely	Normal	Equal to or less than fourfold of the maternal titer at delivery**	NA	NA	No evaluation is recommended
Unlikely	Normal	Equal to or less than fourfold of the maternal titer at delivery***	NA	NA	

**And one of the following: mother was not treated (inadequately or not documented), mother was treated with erythromycin or a non-penicillin G regimen, mother with an adequate treatment but started <30 days before delivery. **And both of the following are true: Mother was treated adequately for infection stage during pregnancy, and treatment was started $\geq$30 days before delivery, and mother has no evidence of reinfection or relapse. ***And both of the following are true: mother's treatment was adequate before pregnancy, and the mother's non-treponemal serologic titer remained low and stable before and ruing pregnancy and at delivery.*

Table 5.
Congenital syphilis possibilities.

Depending of the congenital syphilis possibilities (confirmed proven or highly probable, possible, less likely, unlikely), different treatment doses can be recommended. Congenital Syphilis possibilities are presented in **Table 5**, treatment is described in the corresponding section.

4.3 Diagnosis

As we previously described, many clinical features are common to these diseases, when suspected laboratory confirmation is expected and required.

4.3.1 C. trachomatis and Neisseria gonorrhea

In the case of CT and Ng, we can speak about the type of technologies for diagnosis: batch testing in a laboratory and point-of-care testing as single tests. Currently, the gold standard for the diagnosis of both diseases is the Nucleic Acid Amplification Tests (NAATs). These tests are designed to amplify nucleic acid sequences that are specific for the organism being detected and do not require viable organisms. These kinds of tests can detect even a single copy of the target DNA or RNA. Most important features of batch testing for CT and Ng are included in **Table 6** [15].

Type	Test	CT	Ng
Batch Testing	Culture	48–72 hours of growth High variability and low sensitivity Not for diagnosis	To be examined at 24 hour interval for ≤72 hours Even the high sensitivity and specificity, a very good transportation is required Not for diagnosis
	Nucleic acid amplification tests (NAATs)	(Common to CT and Ng) Gold standard for diagnosis Can detect CT and Ng in: Endocervical swabs from women, Urethral swabs from men, Urine from both men and women	
		CT Commercial NAATs are not known to cross-react with DNA from other bacteria in humans	Ng Some NAATs might cross-react with nongonococcal Neisseria species
	Nucleic acid hybridization (Nucleic Acid Probe) Tests	These tests can detect both pathogens in a single specimen. These tests do not differentiate between the 2 organisms, when positive tests for each organism are needed Advantage: store and transport have a maximum of 7 days without refrigeration	
	Serology tests	Should not be used for screening	A serologic screening or diagnostic assay is not available

Table 6.
Batch testing diagnostic tests for CT and ng.

In the case of CT, point-of-care-tests can be performed within 30-minute delivering qualitative results. For Ng, the current point-of-care test is the Gram stain, this is mostly used in men (urethral exudates); in the case of women, the Gram stain has low sensitivity; therefore, it is not recommended in women.

4.3.1.1 C. trachomatis diagnostic considerations among infants and children

NAATs can be used to test vaginal and urine specimens from girls and urine in boys. There are not enough data about using NAATs for specimens from extragenital sites; nevertheless, there is no evidence supporting that NAAT performance would differ from that among adults. Because of the implications, only validated NAAT tests must be used for diagnosing CT in extragenital sites.

4.3.1.2 Neisseria gonorrhea diagnostic considerations among infants and children

Culture and NAATs can be used to test urogenital and extragenital sites in children. Same as CT, only validated NAAT tests must be used for the diagnosis of Ng in samples coming from extragenital sites. It will be very important to take into account the potential cross-reaction with non-gonococcal Neisseria (i.e., *Neisseria meningitidis, N. sicca, Neisseria lactamica, N. cinerea*) and other commensals (*Moraxella catarrhalis*) for an adequate interpretation of the results.

Gram stains are not recommended in prepuberal children for diagnosis, must NOT be used. In the case of disseminated Ng, culture and antimicrobial susceptibility testing should be obtained from the relevant clinical sites.

4.3.2 Trichomonas vaginalis

Even wet-mount microscopy has been used as the preferred diagnostic test for Trichomonas vaginalis, it is true that with the development of more highly sensitive and specific molecular tests, now the best option is NAATs (98.3% and 99.6%, respectively). Reliable samples include endocervical and vaginal swabs collected by clinicians, female urine specimens, and liquid Pap smear specimens [3].

4.3.3 Syphilis

Darkfield examinations and molecular testes for detecting Tp are the definitive methods for early syphilis and congenital syphilis diagnosis. These tests can be done from material collected directly from the lesion exudate or tissue. Commercial NAATs are not available; nevertheless, some laboratories can provide developed and validated PCR tests.

For a presumptive diagnosis of Syphilis, two types of tests are required:

A Non-treponemal test:

- VDRL (venereal disease research laboratory)

OR

- Rapid plasma reagin (RPR)

AND

A Treponemal test.

Diagnosis of syphilis can start either with a non-treponemal or a treponemal test.

When the first test is a non-treponemal one, confirmation with a treponemal test is always required due to the multiple medical conditions that could result in a false-positive nontreponemal test; some of these are HIV, autoimmune conditions, vaccines, injecting drug use, pregnancy, and older age. Nontreponemal test antibody titers are useful for monitoring treatment response.

If diagnosis of syphilis is established starting with a treponemal test, a quantitative non-treponemal test will be needed for patient management decisions. If non-treponemal test is negative, then the treponemal assay needs to be repeated, this should be different from the one used for initial testing.

Flow of non-treponemal and treponemal tests for decision-making is presented in **Figure 1**.

4.4 Treatment

An important characteristic of these pathogens is the presence of available treatment; nevertheless, antibiotic resistances are becoming a bigger issue every day for Ng. In the case of CT, event with available treatment, many cases are asymptomatic; therefore, available treatment is covering this public health issue partially. Special

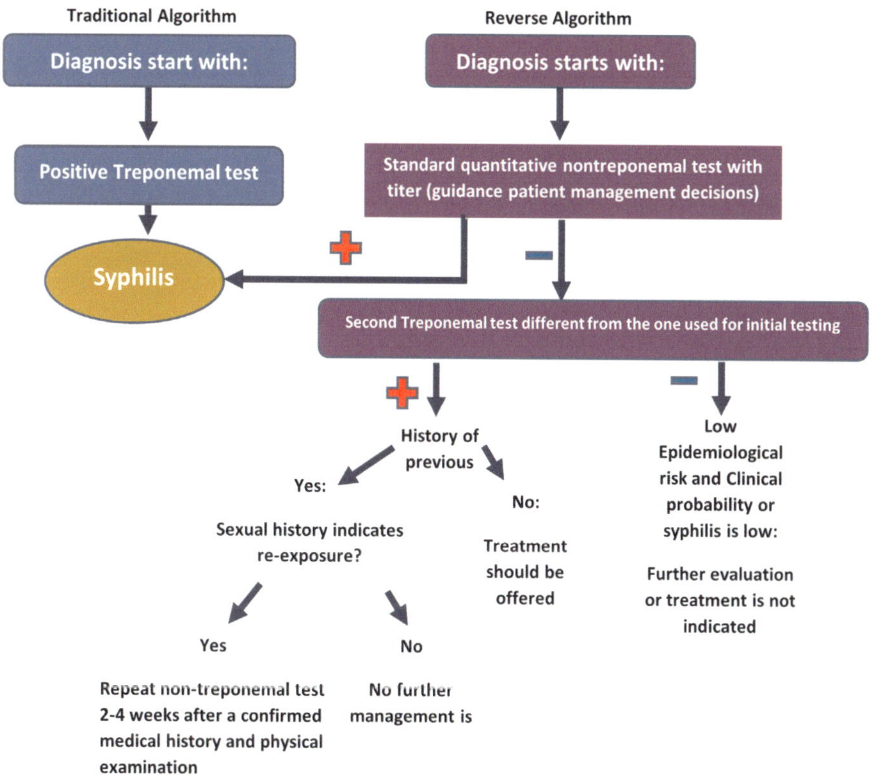

Figure 1.
Traditional and reverse algorithms for syphilis diagnosis.

considerations for pediatrics must be taken into account mostly for Gonorrhea. In **Table 7**, we are presenting the current treatment guidelines per each pathogen [2, 16].

5. Sexual abuse and bacterial sexually transmitted diseases in pediatrics

Sexual abuse should be considered a cause of chlamydial infection among infants and children. Important note: Perinatally transmitted C. trachomatis infection of the nasopharynx, urogenital tract, and rectum can persist for 2–3 years, which is also the most frequent cause of Ng infection in infants and children. If vaginitis is present in preadolescent girls, Ng must be suspected. Nevertheless, pelvic inflammatory disease is less common after vaginal infection in preadolescents. With this finding, Ng must be suspected and tested. Anorectal and pharyngeal infections with Ng in children are frequently asymptomatic; if suspected, samples from these sites must be tested.

Infants and children aged ≥1 month with primary, secondary, or latent syphilis need interdisciplinary treatment including a general pediatrician, a pediatric infectious disease specialist, pediatric psychologist, and social work, which must be evaluated for sexual abuse, and child protective services must be alerted based on local laws.

In the adolescent population, survivors of sexual assault must be examined by experienced clinicians, the obtention of genital or other specimens has to be decided individually and in accordance with local laws. Tv, Ng, and CT are the most common diagnosed pathogens. NAATs for CT and Ng at the site of penetration and for Tv in

Treatment	CT	Ng	Tp	Tv
Affected patient	Neonates: Oral erythromycin base or ethyl succinate 50 mg/kg body weight/day divided into 4 doses daily for 14 days Chlamydial Pneumonia Among Infants: oral erythromycin base or ethyl succinate 50 mg/kg body weight/day orally divided into 4 doses daily for 14 days (alternative regimen: oral azithromycin suspension 20 mg/kg/day, 1 dose daily for 3 days) Infants and children: Weighing <45 kg: Erythromycin base or ethyl succinate 50 mg/kg body weight/day orally divided into 4 doses daily for 14 days Weighing ≥45 kg but aged <8 years: Azithromycin 1 g orally in a single dose Children aged ≥8 years: Azithromycin 1 g orally in a single dose OR Doxycycline 100 mg orally 2 times/day for 7 day Adolescents and Adults: Oral Doxycycline 100 mg 2 times per day for 7 days Alternative regimens: Oral Azithromycin 1 g, single dose OR Oral Levofloxacin 500 mg once daily for 7 days Pregnancy: Oral Azithromycin 1 g,	Adult and Adolescents: Uncomplicated Gonococcal Infection of the Cervix, Urethra, or Rectum: Ceftriaxone 500 mg Intramuscular (IM) in a single dose for persons weighing < 150 kg (If ≥150 kg, 1 g ceftriaxone). Alternatives if ceftriaxone is not available: Gentamicin 240 mg IM in a single dose plus Azithromycin 2 g orally in a single dose OR Cefixime 800 mg orally in a single dose Uncomplicated gonococcal infection of the pharynx: Ceftriaxone 500 mg IM in a single dose for persons weighing <150 kg (if ≥150 kg, 1 g ceftriaxone). Gonococcal Conjunctivitis Ceftriaxone 1 g IM in a single dose (one time lavage of the infected eye with saline solution must be considered) Gonococcal-Related Arthritis and Arthritis-Dermatitis Syndrome Ceftriaxone 1 g IM or IV every 24 hours (alternative regimen: Alternative Regimens Cefotaxime 1 g IV every 8 hours or Ceftizoxime 1 g every 8 hours) Neonates, Infants and Children Ophthalmia Neonatorum PREVENTION: Erythromycin 0.5% ophthalmic ointment in each eye in a single application at birth Ophthalmia Neonatorum TREATMENT: Ceftriaxone 25–50 mg/kg body weight IV or IM in a single dose, not to exceed 250 mg	Parenteral Penicillin G (dosage and length of the treatment depend on the stage and clinical manifestations) Congenital Syphilis: Confirmed or highly probable: Aqueous crystalline penicillin G 100,000–150,000 units/kg/body weight per day, administered as 50,000 units/kg/body weight per dose IV every 12 hours during the first 7 days of life and every 8 hours thereafter for a total of 10 days OR Procaine penicillin G 50,000 units/kg/body weight per dose IM in a single daily dose for 10 days Possible: Same as confirmed with and additional option of Benzathine penicillin G 50,000 units/kg body weight/dose IM in a single dose Less Likely and unlikely: Benzathine penicillin G, same doses as possible. Infants and children: Benzathine penicillin G 50,000 units/kg body weight IM, up to the adult dose of 2.4 million units in a single dose Adults: Primary, Secondary and Early latent: Benzathine penicillin G 2.4 million units IM in a single dose Late latent: Benzathine penicillin G 7.2 million units total, administered as 3 doses of 2.4 million units IM each at 1-week intervals Tertiary: Benzathine penicillin G 7.2	Women: Metronidazole 500 mg orally 2 times/day for 7 days Men: Metronidazole 2 g orally in a single dose Alternative regimen for women and men: Tinidazole 2 g orally in a single dose

DOI: http://dx.doi.org/10.5772/intechopen.107991

Treatment	CT	Ng	Tp	Tv
	single dose (alternative: oral Amoxicillin 500 mg 3 times a day for 7 days	Disseminated Gonococcal Infection Among Neonates: Ceftriaxone 25–50 mg/kg body weight/day IV or IM in a single daily dose for 7 days, with a duration of 10–14 days if meningitis is documented OR Cefotaxime 25 mg/kg body weight/day IV or IM every 12 hours for 7 days, with a duration of 10–14 days if meningitis is documented Neonates without signs of gonococcal infection: Ceftriaxone 20–50 mg/kg body weight IV or IM in a single dose, maximum 250 mg Uncomplicated Gonococcal Vulvovaginitis, Cervicitis, Urethritis, Pharyngitis, or Proctitis Among Infants and Children: Weighing ≤45 kg: Ceftriaxone 25–50 mg/kg body weight IV or IM in a single dose, not to exceed 250 mg IM Weighing >45 kg: same as adults Bacteremia or Arthritis Among Children: Weighing ≤45 kg: Ceftriaxone 50 mg/kg body weight (maximum dose: 2 g) IM or IV in a single dose daily every 24 hours for 7 days Weighing >45 kg: Ceftriaxone 1 g IM or IV in a single dose daily every 24 hours for 7 days	million units total, administered as 3 doses of 2.4 million units IM each at 1-week intervals	
Sex partners	Sex partners should receive treatment if they had sexual contact with the partner during the 60 days preceding	Sex partners: current or the most recent must be treated: Cefixime 800 mg as a single dose	Contact <90 days before the diagnosis, needs treatment for early syphilis, even if serologic test is	Concurrent treatment of all sexual partners is crucial for preventing reinfections.

Treatment	CT	Ng	Tp	Tv
	the patient's onset of symptoms or chlamydia diagnosis. The most recent sex partner should be treated.	If CT has not been excluded, a single dose of doxycycline 100 mg 2 times/day for 7 days must be added.	negative Contact >90 days before diagnosis and serological tests are not immediately available, treatment for early syphilis is needed. If serological test is negative treatment is not needed Partners among populations with high syphilis rates Long-term sex partners of persons with latent syphilis	Partners should abstain from intercourse until they and their sex partners have been treated and any symptoms have resolved.
Highlights	In neonates: An association between oral erythromycin and azithromycin and infantile hypertrophic pyloric stenosis (IHPS) has been reported among infants aged <6 weeks. IHPS signs and symptoms must be followed-up Persons treated for chlamydia should be instructed to abstain from sexual intercourse for 7 days after single-dose therapy or until completion of a 7-day regimen and resolution of symptoms if present (Transmission reduction) Patients should abstain from sexual intercourse until all of their sex partners have been treated. Persons who receive a diagnosis of chlamydia should be tested for HIV, gonorrhea, and syphilis.	In neonates, ceftriaxone must be administered cautiously: In the presence of hyperbilirubinemia (especially premature newborns) If IV calcium is necessary to be administered simultaneously, an appropriate alternative is cefotaxime 100 mg/kg body weight IV or IM, single dose. In any case and in any age, if chlamydial infection has not been excluded, treatment for chlamydia must be added.	Jarisch-Herxheimer Reaction: acute febrile reaction frequently accompanied by headache, myalgia, and fever within 24 hours after treatment initiation. Antipyretics can be used. DO NOT DELAY TREATMENT BECAUSE OF THE REACTION In pediatric age, sexual abuse must be investigated in all cases	Recurrent Tv can result from treatment failure, lack of adherence, or reinfection from an untreated sex partner. Nitroimidazole resistant Tv is concerning due to few alternatives to standard therapy. Metronidazole resistance occurs in 4–10% of cases, and tinidazole apparently around 1%

Table 7.
Treatment for the patient and sexual partners per pathogen with some highlights.

urine or vaginal specimen are recommended. Empiric antimicrobial regimens must be started, for women must include Ceftriaxone 500 mg IM in a single dose, Doxycycline 100 mg two times per day orally for 7 days and metronidazole 500 mg two times per day orally for 7 days. In men, ceftriaxone and doxycycline are recommended with the same doses than women. For persons weighing ≥150 kg, 1 g of ceftriaxone should be administered.

In children, the most important factors that must lead a clinician to evaluate sexually transmitted diseases due to sexual abuse include evidence of penetration or healed penetrative injury to the genitals, anus, or oropharynx, abuse is reported, the child has a relative or another person in his/her same environment with a sexually transmitted disease, signs or symptoms such as vaginal discharge or pain, genital itching or odor, urinary symptoms, or genital lesions or ulcers.

Conflict of interest

Diana Leticia Coronel Martinez is an employee of Sanofi.

Author details

Diana Leticia Coronel Martínez[1]* and Luis Augusto Moya Barquín[2]

1 Pediatric Resuscitation Advanced Group, Mexico City, Mexico

2 Pediatric Critical Care Unit at San Juan de Dios of Guatemala General Hospital, San Carlos of Guatemala University, Mexico

*Address all correspondence to: dianacoronel75@gmail.com

References

[1] Rowley J, Vander Hoorn S, Korenromp E, et al. Chlamydia, gonorrhoea, trichomoniasis and syphilis: Global prevalence and incidence estimates, 2016. Bulletin of the World Health Organization. 2019; **97**(8):548-562P. DOI: 10.2471/BLT.18.228486

[2] Sexually Transmitted Disease Surveillance 2020. Centers of Disease Control and Prevention [Internet]. 2022. Available from: https://www.cdc.gov/std/statistics/2020/default.htm [Accessed: June 23, 2022]

[3] Trichomoniasis. Centers of Disease Control and Prevention [Internet]. 2021. Available from: https://www.cdc.gov/std/trichomonas/stats.htm [Accessed: June 23, 2022]

[4] Witkin SS, Minis E, Athanasiou A, Leizer J, Linhares IM. Chlamydia trachomatis: The persistent pathogen. Clinical and Vaccine Immunology. 2017; **24**(10):e00203-e00217. DOI: 10.1128/CVI.00203-17

[5] Lane AB, Decker CF. Chlamydia trachomatis infections. Disease-a-Month. 2016;**62**(8):269-273. DOI: 10.1016/j.disamonth.2016.03.010

[6] Klöckner A, Bühl H, Violler P, Henrichfreise B. Deconstructing the chlamydia Cell Wall. In: Häcker G, editor. Biology of Chlamydia. Switzerland: Springer Nature; 2018. pp. 2-26. DOI: 10.1007/978-3-319-71232-1

[7] Häcker G. Preface. Replace the entirety of this text with your references. In: Häcker G, editor. Biology of Chlamydia. Switzerland: Springer Nature; 2018. pp. v-vii. DOI: 10.1007/978-3-319-71232-1

[8] Hook EW 3rd, Kirkcaldy RD. A brief history of evolving diagnostics and therapy for gonorrhea: Lessons learned. Clinical Infectious Diseases. 2018;**67**(8): 1294-1299. DOI: 10.1093/cid/ciy271

[9] Unemo M, Seifert HS, Hook EW 3rd, Hawkes S, Ndowa F, Dillon JR. Gonorrhoea. Nature Reviews. Disease Primers. 2019;**5**(1):79. DOI: 10.1038/s41572-019-0128-6

[10] Quillin SJ, Seifert HS. Neisseria gonorrhoeae host adaptation and pathogenesis. Nature Reviews. Microbiology. 2018;**16**(4):226-240. DOI: 10.1038/nrmicro.2017.169

[11] Smajs D, Norris SJ, Weinstock GM. Genetic diversity in Treponema pallidum: Implications for pathogenesis, evolution and molecular diagnostics of syphilis and yaws. Infection, Genetics and Evolution. 2012;**12**:191-202

[12] Peeling RW, Mabey D, Kamb ML, Chen XS, Radolf JD, Benzaken AS. Syphilis. Nature Reviews. Disease Primers. 2017;**3**:17073. DOI: 10.1038/nrdp.2017.73

[13] Edwards T, Burke P, Smalley H, Hobbs G. Trichomonas vaginalis: Clinical relevance, pathogenicity and diagnosis. Critical Reviews in Microbiology. 2016; **42**(3):406-417. DOI: 10.3109/1040841X.2014.958050

[14] Centers for Disease Control and Prevention. Screening tests to detect chlamydia trachomatis and Neisseria gonorrhoeae infections — 2002. MMWR. 2002;**51**(RR-15):1-38

[15] Workowski KA, Bachmann LH, Chan PA, et al. Sexually transmitted infections treatment guidelines, 2021. MMWR - Recommendations and

Reports. 2021;**70**(4):1-187.
DOI: 10.15585/mmwr.rr7004a1

[16] IntechOpen Book Chapter Layout uses the numbered citation method for reference formatting, with sequential numbering in the text, and respective ordering in a list at the end of the paper

Chapter 4

False-Positive Serologic Reactions for Syphilis

Nikolay Potekaev, Olga Zhukova and Irina Khamaganova

Abstract

The epidemiologic situation of syphilitic infection warrants attention to diagnostic methods. Nontreponemal tests (rapid plasma regain, Venereal Disease Research Laboratory) are less reliable, as there are certain situations when false-positive reactions for syphilis antibodies may appear. Variable examinations were performed and proved that it was necessary to assess the titer of antibodies, as well as confirmation of the diagnosis by treponemal tests (fluorescent treponemal antibody, treponema pallidum hemagglutination assay, enzyme immunoassay, Western blot), were obligatory. In recent decades, new methods were elaborated (e.g., BioPlex total screen, tests with β2-GPI-dependent anticardiolipin antibody, the ARCHITECT syphilis treponema pallidum chemiluminescent immunoassay, the Elecsys immunoassay (Roche Diagnostics)). We present the review of publications on syphilis serologic diagnostics and present our own research. We did not find any mention of a false-positive test in atopic dermatitis and present a case of false-positive reactions for syphilis in such patients.

Keywords: syphilis, serologic diagnostic, nontreponemal tests, treponemal tests, false-positive serologic reactions

1. Introduction

The incidence of syphilis has been increasing from the end of twentieth century—early 2000s [1, 2], warranting attention to diagnostic methods. Now we have serious problems in serologic diagnostic of different clinical forms of syphilis, including those of atypical duration, cardiovascular syphilis, neurosyphilis, congenital syphilis, latent forms, etc. Nontreponemal tests (rapid plasma regain, Venereal Disease Research Laboratory) are less reliable as there are certain situations when false-positive reactions for syphilis antibodies may appear. Variable examinations were performed and proved that it was necessary to assess the titer of antibodies, as well as confirmation of the diagnosis by treponemal tests (fluorescent treponemal antibody, treponema pallidum hemagglutination assay, enzyme immunoassay, Western blot), were obligatory. In recent decades, new methods were elaborated (e.g., BioPlex total screen, tests with β2-GPI-dependent anticardiolipin antibody, the ARCHITECT syphilis treponema pallidum chemiluminescent immunoassay, the Elecsys immunoassay (Roche Diagnostics)) [3–15] to exclude false-positive and false-negative reactions. Syphilis as the "great imitator" may be presented by a variety of clinical signs and symptoms of infection that can be easily confused with other diseases [16–18]. But in spite of miscellaneous investigations, complexities in the diagnosis of syphilis continue to challenge clinicians [19–24]. For instance, discordant maternal reverse-sequence serology is still a problem in diagnosis of congenital syphilis [25, 26]. We analyzed the papers presented in PUB MED. By the end of December 2021, the search query "False-positive reactions for syphilis" gave 743 publications. We included the papers published in English from January 2010 till the end of December 2021. We excluded the papers publicized earlier than in 2010, written in other languages than English, and those which had nothing to do with our demand "False-positive tests for syphilis". So, we analyzed 88 publications and presented our own research. We did not find any mention of false-positive tests in atopic dermatitis and present a case of false-positive reactions for syphilis in such patients.

2. Clinical situations with false-positive syphilis reactions

A substantial problem is presented now by discordant serologic reactions for syphilis in different clinical situations [27–31]. Huh et al. [32] pointed to the growth of false-positive reactions in syphilis screening assays and proved that the reverse algorithm using Automated Mediace Treponema pallidum latex agglutination (TPLA) as a screening serologic test is preferred over rapid plasma reagin (RPR) assays [32, 33]. Furthermore, the biological false-positive Venereal Disease Research Laboratory (VDRL)—cerebrospinal fluid test is often used in cases when patients are examined without a previous serological diagnosis of syphilis [20]. Palamar et al. retrospectively explored the serologic blood sample and microbiological culture media analysis results of all cornea donors. False-positive serologic results among cornea donors were high [34], which underlines the importance of the improvement of serologic diagnostic in this field. Last year, different clinical situations confirmed the actual need for further serologic investigations [24, 35–37].

Dunseth et al. underlined the necessity of differentiation between analytical false-positive results of lues tests from clinical false-positive results. A positive syphilis IgG screen with negative RPR and T. pallidum particle agglutination assay (TP-PA) confirmatory testing could be considered an analytical false-positive. A positive syphilis IgG with positive TP-PA and negative RPR might be an analytical false-positive due to cross-reacting antibodies or analytical true-positive result in late/latent syphilis or past/treated syphilis with persistent anti-syphilis IgG. Nontreponemal tests may show false-positive screens due to a variety of reasons [38]. Ishihara et al. presented a retrospective study of patients tested for syphilis in a tertiary academic hospital. Among 94,462 subjects, 588 patients had false-positive tests (0.62%). Such cases were noted in patients aged over 60 years, with a history of malignancy and autoimmune diseases [36]. But the false-positive tests for syphilis were noted in children as well [37]. Over all 90% of biologically false-positive reactions are low titer (≤1:4), but (1%) are high-titer (≥1:32) [24]. Such reactions are categorized as either acute (occurring for less than 6 months) or chronic [19, 28]. Acute false-positive reactions are noted in febrile illnesses, immunizations, and pregnancy [29–31, 38–40]. For example, Nwosu et al. examined 2156 women, VDRL was positive in 15 cases (0.70%). Confirmatory T. pallidum hemagglutination assay was positive in 4 of the 15 cases, giving an overall prevalence of 0.19% and a false-positive rate of 73.3%. There was no significant difference in the prevalence of syphilis in relation to maternal age and parity ($P > 0.05$) [41].

As for chronic false-positive reactions, they can be noted in such clinical cases as hepatitis C virus (HCV) infection, intravenous drug use, malignancy, older age, malaria, Chagas disease, tuberculosis, leprosy, and connective tissue diseases [28]. Besides, false-positive test is a characteristic clinical sign in patients with systemic lupus erythematosus [42, 43]. It is proved now that false-positive results of serologic reactions for syphilis may be caused by HCV [44]. Some investigations showed that different types of cryoglobulinemia might be accompanied by acute or chronic false-positive reactions [45].

Further investigation demonstrated that racial and environmental factors, as well as immuno-chromatographic dual syphilis rapid testing may affect [46], and that can be used in clinical practice.

Augenbraun et al. concluded that HCV infection was associated with certain mechanisms changing the immune function including alterations in serological reactions results. He underlined as well that women with HCV were more likely to have biological false-positive syphilis tests than women without HCV [47].

Furthermore, Bright et al. noted that false-positive reactions might be marked in patients treated with pooled human immunoglobulin G infusions [48].

In 2014, Liu et al. named diseases that had not been previously reported to be associated with the classical biological false-positive reaction, such as false-labor, megaloblastic anemias, aplastic anemias, redundant prepuce, congenital malformation of heart, and salpingitis [49].

Nowadays the significance of sera with isolated reactive treponemal chemiluminescence immunoassay (IRTCIA) results is being discussed. It is known that as a rule, women have this phenotype more commonly than men. Bopage et al. presented the results of the examination 19/63 (30.1%) subjects with the IRTCIA phenotype, which were positive in the line immunoblot assay (LIA). It was marked that women were substantially less likely to have definitive results (positive or negative) than men ($p = 0.015$). And women who were pregnant less likely than nonpregnant women to have a negative LIA result (OR 0.57; $p = 0.03$). Record review of 22 different women with IRTCIA reactivity allowed to reveal that 2/22 (9.1%) had HIV and previous syphilis infection, 15/22 (68.2%) were pregnant, and 3 (13.6%) had autoimmune disease [50].

McGready et al. emphasized that the potential impact of false-positive tests should be considered in HIV- positives [51]. And vice versa, false-negative lues tests are noted in HIV- positives subjects [52].

Cantor et al. analyzed a 2004 systematic review of studies of syphilis screening effectiveness, test accuracy, and screening harms in nonpregnant women and adolescents. It was proved that screening HIV-positive men or men who have sex with men (MSM) for syphilis every 3 months is associated with improved syphilis detection [53].

Today there are no doubts that HIV-positive patients [54, 55], MSM, and transgender women are at high risk of acquiring syphilis and HIV infection [56].

The results presented by Kalou et al. indicate that this assay could have a significant impact on the simultaneous screening of HIV and syphilis using a single test device for high-risk populations or pregnant women needing timely care and treatment [57]. Shakya et al. also underlined the importance of simultaneous diagnosis of HIV and syphilis [58].

Grégoire et al. presented the results of the examination of donors who had false-positive tests for HIV, HBV, HCV, or syphilis. Rates of second false-positive results were compared by year of deferral, transmissible disease marker, gender, age, donor status (new or repeat), and testing platform (same or different) both at qualification for re-entry and afterward. The risk, when analyzed by multivariate analyses, of a second deferral for a false-positive result, both at qualification and 3 years after reentry, was lower for donors deferred on a different platform; this risk was higher for HIV, HCV and syphilis than for HBV and for new donors if tested on the same platform [59]. The importance of thorough examination of HIV subjects with false-positive reactions for syphilis was marked in other investigations as well [60, 61].

Sandes et al. presented the results of analyses of the positive and false-positive tests of treponemal and nontreponemal tests in blood donors and found out that older donors and donors with lower education levels were associated with a higher risk of positivity for syphilis [62].

3. Modern serologic diagnostic

The World Health Organization recommendations of screening for syphilis in a low prevalence population of blood donors using enzyme-linked immune-sorbent assay (ELISA) may be adopted for usage in transfusion services that have the facility of ELISA [63].

On the other hand, the current screening of deceased organ donors by RPR yields a significant number of false-positive results [64].

And vice versa, in patients with positive Lyme screening and negative confirmatory testing, the performance of lues serology should be considered [29, 65, 66].

Park et al. [67], Hoover and Radolf [68], Dassah et al. emphasized the importance of the improvement of the serologic diagnostic [69]. Overall, nontreponemal tests were less sensitive than treponema-specific tests [70].

Nah et al. investigated the efficacy of traditional and reverse syphilis diagnostic algorithms during general health checkups. In total, 1000 blood specimens were obtained from 908 men and 92 women. As a result, the reverse screening algorithm could detect the subjects with possible latent syphilis who were not detected by the traditional algorithm [71].

Rourk and Litwin investigated the recently FDA cleared BioPlex 2200 syphilis total screen and automated RPR assay for the detection of total (IgG/IgM) treponemal and nontreponemal antibodies in the reverse syphilis algorithm. They concluded that the addition of the detection of treponemal IgM antibodies to the IgG/IgM screen had not significantly affected the sensitivity and specificity compared to the original IgG screen. But the addition of the comparable BioPlex RPR assay to the instrumentation significantly reduced the overall labor of syphilis screening and confirmation [72].

Yen-Lieberman et al. noted that regardless of the method, laboratories should develop approaches to identify analytical false-positive results wherever possible [73].

The syphilis testing may be affected by different racial and environmental factors [46], which is necessary to keep in mind at the estimation of serologic results.

Zhou et al. marked a high correlation between electrochemiluminescence immunoassay analyzer and chemiluminescent magnetic microparticle immunoassay. Both had high sensitivity and specificity [74].

The appearance of β2-GPI-dependent anticardiolipin antibody and its association with blood coagulation have been investigated in subjects with classical biological false-positive syphilis reactions. Subjects with false-positive tests for syphilis appeared to be more prone to blood coagulation disorders than syphilis patients, and these autoantibodies may impact the intrinsic coagulation cascade in cases of false-positive reactions, similar to presumed antiphospholipid antibody syndrome patients [75].

Considering the importance of the diagnosis of syphilis, antibodies to T. pallidum in serum samples should be retested by the improved ELISA method to avoid false-positive results [76]. Different reverse syphilis testing algorithms were proposed [77].

While in screening populations, discrepancies between chemiluminescent microparticle immunoassay and treponema pallidum particle agglutination results are quite prevalent, confirmation by immunoblot assay may be useful [78]. The ARCHITECT syphilis treponema pallidum chemiluminescent immunoassay accurately diagnoses current or past syphilis in pregnancy [79].

The Elecsys immunoassay (Roche Diagnostics) yielded no false-negative results and fewer false-positive results, compared to the other tests [80]. However, Li et al. underlined that the Elecsys® syphilis assay might be confirmed by other treponemal immunoassays [81].

Enders et al. noted that the specificity of the Elecsys syphilis assay in patients with other infections had been 100%; no false-positive samples had been identified [82].

Simčič and Potočnik supported the European Center for Disease Prevention and Control algorithm in the serodiagnosis of syphilis in high-prevalence populations and the use of nontreponemal serology to monitor the response to treatment [83].

Song et al. evaluated diagnostic methods for revealing syphilis in children. False-positive tests for syphilis were higher in the children's group than in the infant's group. The high false-positive rate of enzyme-linked immuno-sorbent assay (ELISA) could be caused by hemolysis. The RPR had low sensitivity in suspected syphilis neonates, and the colloidal gold test (SYP) was suitable for emergency treatment. The treponema pallidum particle agglutination test (TPPA) was fit for the diagnosis of syphilis [84].

It is obvious that further investigations are necessary, and different forms of syphilis need a specific complex of serologic reactions.

4. Own research

Since January 2014 till December 2021, we examined nine patients with false-positive serologic tests for syphilis, aged 48—79. They had no medical documentation with any mentioning of syphilis was presented. They denied syphilitic infection in the past. Three patients were diagnosed with breast cancer, three patients were diagnosed with ovarian cancer, two patients were diagnosed with lupus erythematosus, and one patient was diagnosed with liver cancer.

A 79-year-old patient with liver cancer suffered from diabetes mellitus and obesity as well. The patient denied syphilitic infection in anamnesis. No clinical signs of syphilis were revealed. He was examined thoroughly, and four times during examination and before the operation the micro-reaction of precipitation with plasma and in activated serum and inactivated serum was false-positive, treponemal tests (reaction of passive hemagglutination, immunoenzyme analysis for treponema pallidum) were negative.

A 49-year-old patient suffering from chronic cholecystitis, a 50-year-old patient suffering from thyroiditis, 51-year-old patient suffering from diabetes mellitus showed false-positive serologic reactions for syphilis during the examination and before the operation for breast cancer showed false- positive micro-reaction of precipitation with plasma and in activated serum and inactivated serum was revealed in these cases, treponemal tests (reaction of passive hemagglutination, immunoenzyme analysis for treponema pallidum) were negative.

A 48-year-old patient, 50-year-old patient, 51-year-old patient had no concomitant diseases, and only after revealing ovarian cancer false-positive micro-reaction of precipitation with plasma and in activated serum and inactivated serum was revealed in these cases, treponemal tests (reaction of passive hemagglutination, immunoenzyme analysis for treponema pallidum) were negative. Repeated studies did not show any changes in serologic reactions.

A 49- and 60-year-old patients with chronic lupus erythematosus showed false-positive reactions for syphilis since their first diagnosis of lupus erythematosus, accordingly 20 and 37 years ago.

As a result of our search, we proved that different clinical situations (cancer, lupus erythematosus) were accompanied by false-positive tests for syphilis, but we did not find any mention of false-positive test in atopic dermatitis (AD). Meanwhile, the disease is not rare in different countries [85–92]. Now, we present the case.

5. Case

A 37-year-old man suffered from AD since the age of 3 months. Most part of his childhood he spent in hospitals due to exacerbations of AD. The treatment included pharmacotherapy and physiotherapy treatment. Usually, hospital courses were accompanied by subsequent spa courses. No seasonality was noted. In adulthood, the patient worked as a software developer, but the exacerbations of atopic dermatitis continued to be frequent. For the past 3 years the micro-reaction of precipitation with plasma and in activated serum and inactivated serum was false-positive, no clinical signs of syphilis were revealed, and treponemal tests (reaction of passive hemagglutination, immunoenzyme analysis for treponema pallidum) were negative. Earlier the patient had passed some childhood infections, and acute respiratory viral infections. The patient denied syphilitic infection in anamnesis. And no medical documentation with any mention of syphilis was presented.

The past 2 weeks' acute inflammation on the skin is noted. The patient suffered from severe itching and insomnia. The face, scalp, neck, trunk, and upper and lower extremities are involved. The skin is dry. The periorbital zone presented moderate swelling and rugosity. The mouth angles are infiltrated (**Figure 1**). The elbow bands and popliteal spaces are lichenificated (**Figure 2**). Polymorphous eruptions with infiltrated erythema, excoriations, and superficial erosions with irregular borders were located on the scalp, neck, trunk, and extremities. Dermographism is persistent white.

The results of blood analysis were within normal limits, except the erythrocyte sedimentation rate, which was 43.

The analysis of AIDS and hepatitis was negative.

The micro-reaction of precipitation with plasma and in activated serum and inactivated serum was negative both with capillary and venous blood. The reaction of passive hemagglutination, immunoenzyme analysis for treponema pallidum) were negative.

So, the patient with severe AD had typical false-positive tests for syphilis, when the nontreponemal test was positive and treponemal tests were negative.

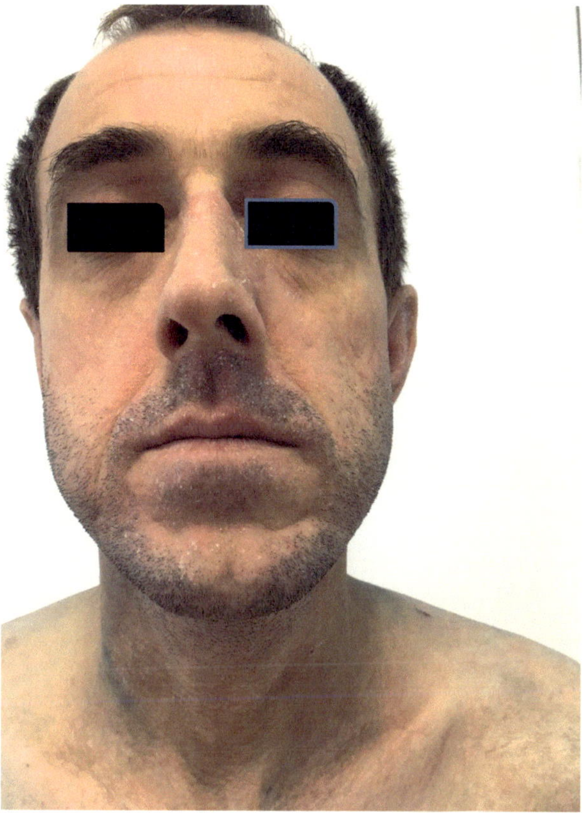

Figure 1.
Lesions on the face.

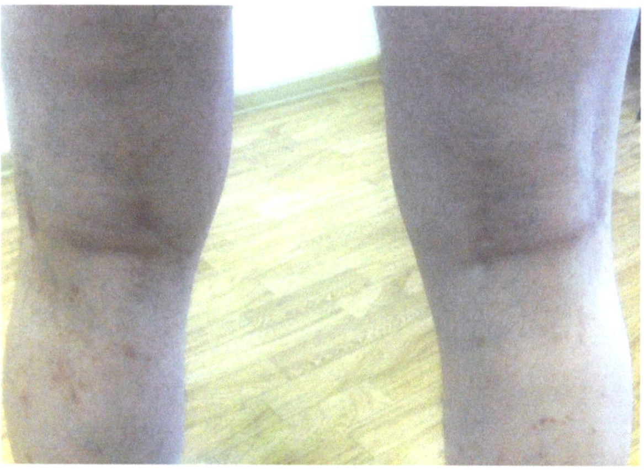

Figure 2.
Lesions in popliteal areas.

6. Conclusion

To summarize, the problem of false-positive tests for syphilis needs a multidisciplinary approach as it may accompany different diseases and the complex diagnostics tests must be upgraded. Chronic inflammation of long duration, immune changes of reactivity may lead to increased production of antibodies to lipids or plasma proteins and false-positive tests for syphilis in a patient with a severe duration of atopic dermatitis.

Author details

Nikolay Potekaev[1,2]*, Olga Zhukova[2] and Irina Khamaganova[3]

1 Moscow Scientific and Practical Center of Dermatovenerology and Cosmetology, Moscow, Russia

2 Department of Skin Diseases and Cosmetology, Pirogov Russian National Research Medical University, Moscow, Russia

3 Department of Skin and Venereal Diseases, Institute of Medicine, RUDN University, Moscow, Russia

*Address all correspondence to: irina.khamaganova@gmail.com

References

[1] Mattei PL, Beachkofsky TM, Gilson RT, Wisco OJ. Syphilis: A reemerging infection. American Family Physician. 2012;**86**(5):433-440

[2] Sethi S, Mewara A, Hallur V, Prasad A, Sharma K, Raj A. Rising trends of syphilis in a tertiary care center in North India. Indian Journal of Sex Transmitted Diseases AIDS. 2015;**36**(2):140-143

[3] Boonchaoy A, Wongchampa P, Hirankarn N, Chaithongwongwatthana S. Performance of chemiluminescent microparticle immunoassay in screening for syphilis in pregnant women from low-prevalence, resource-limited setting. Journal of Medical Association Thailand. 2016;**99**(2):119-124

[4] Cantor A, Nelson HD, Daeges M, Pappas M. Screening for Syphilis in Nonpregnant Adolescents and Adults: Systematic Review to Update the 2004 U.S. Preventive Services Task Force Recommendation [Internet]. Evidence Syntheses. 2016;**2016**:136

[5] Dlamini NR, Phili R, Connolly C. Evaluation of rapid syphilis tests in KwaZulu-Natal. Journal of Clinical Laboratory Analysis. 2014;**28**(1):77-81

[6] Donkers A, Levy HR, Letens-van VA. Syphilis detection using the Siemens ADVIA centaur syphilis treponemal assay. Clinica Chimica Acta. 2014;**433**:84-87

[7] Li D, Chen Z, Tao C. Comparison of three syphilis algorithms in West China. Clinica Chimica Acta. 2019;**488**:76-80

[8] Obafemi OA, Wendel KA, Anderson TS, Scott TE, Rowan SE, Travanty EA, et al. Rapid syphilis testing for men who have sex with men in outreach settings: Evaluation of test performance and impact on time to treatment. Sexually Transmitted Diseases. 2019;**46**(3):191-195. DOI: 10.1097/OLQ.0000000000000932

[9] Park BG, Yoon JG, Rim JH, Lee A, Kim HS. Comparison of six automated Treponema-specific antibody assays. Journal of Clinical Microbiology. 2016;**54**(1):163-167

[10] Richards J, Matthias J, Baker C, Wilson C, Peterman TA, Brown CP, et al. Evaluation of rapid syphilis testing using the syphilis health check in Florida, 2015-2016. Florida Public Health Review. 2019;**16**:13

[11] Sarkodie F, Ullum H, Owusu-Dabo E, Owusu-Ofori S, Owusu-Ofori A, Hassall O. A novel strategy for screening blood donors for syphilis at Komfo Anokye teaching hospital, Ghana. Transfusion Medicine. 2016;**26**(1).63-66

[12] Shimelis T, Tadesse E. The diagnostic performance evaluation of the SD BIOLINE HIV/syphilis duo rapid test in southern Ethiopia: A cross-sectional study. BMJ Open. 2015;**5**(4):e007371

[13] Xu M, Xie Y, Jiang C, Xiao Y, Kuang X, Zhao F, et al. A novel ELISA using a recombinant outer membrane protein, rTp0663, as the antigen for serological diagnosis of syphilis. International Journal of Infectious Diseases. 2016;**43**:51-57

[14] Zhiyan L, Meiling W, Ping L, Jinhua D, Zhenlin Y, Zhenru F. Consistency between Treponema pallidum particle agglutination assay and Architect chemiluminescent

microparticle immunoassay and characterization of inconsistent samples. Journal of Clinical Laboratory Analysis. 2015;**29**(4):281-284

[15] Zhuang YH, Liu H, Tang J, Wang YZ, Zheng XH, Gong Y, et al. Screening for syphilis with dual algorithms: Analysis of discordant and concordant serology results in a population with a low prevalence of syphilis. Journal of the European Academy of Dermatology and Venereology. 2019;**33**(1):178-184

[16] Ngan W, Chiu PK, Chung HY. Primary Sjogren syndrome masquerading as a false-positive venereal disease research laboratory and fluorescent treponemal antibody absorption test in an elderly woman. Journal of the American Geriatrics Society. 2014;**62**(9):1817-1818. DOI: 10.1111/jgs.13013

[17] Shi H, Luo W, Li W, Shen C, Liu X, Liu F, et al. Serologic false-positive reactions for syphilis in children of allergic purpura. Clinical Chemistry and Laboratory Medicine. 2015;**53**(9):e223-e225. DOI: 10.1515/cclm-2014-0489

[18] Soreng K, Levy R, Fakile Y. Serologic testing for syphilis: Benefits and challenges of a reverse algorithm. Clinical Microbiology Newsletter. 2014;**36**(24):195-202. DOI: 10.1016/j.clinmicnews.2014.12.001

[19] Harman LE, Margo CE, Roetzheim RG. Uveitis: The collaborative diagnostic evaluation. American Family Physician. 2014;**90**(10):711-716

[20] Morshed MG, Singh AE. Recent trends in the serologic diagnosis of syphilis. Clinical and Vaccine Immunology. 2015;**22**(2):137-147

[21] Patriquin G, LeBlanc J, Heinstein C, Roberts C, Lindsay R, Hatchette TF. Cross-reactivity between Lyme and syphilis screening assays: Lyme disease does not cause false-positive syphilis screens. Diagnostic Microbiology and Infectious Disease. 2016;**84**(3):184-186

[22] Cantor AG, Pappas M, Daeges M, Nelson HD. Screening for syphilis: Updated evidence report and systematic review for the US preventive services task force. Screening for syphilis: Updated evidence report and systematic review for the US preventive services task force. Journal of the American Medical Association. 2016;**315**(21):2328-2337. DOI: 10.1001/jama.2016.4114

[23] Negash M, Wondmagegn T, Geremew D. Comparison of RPR and ELISA with TPHA for the diagnosis of syphilis: Implication for updating syphilis point-of-care tests in Ethiopia. Journal of Immunology Research. 2018;**2018**:2978419

[24] Matthias J, Klingler EJ, Schillinger JA, Keller G, Wilson C, Peterman TA. Frequency and characteristics of biological false-positive test results for syphilis reported in Florida and New York City, USA, 2013 to 2017. Journal of Clinical Microbiology. 2019;**57**(11):e00898

[25] Patel NU, Oussedik E, Landis ET, Strowd LC. Early congenital syphilis: Recognising symptoms of an increasingly prevalent disease. Journal of Cutaneous Medical Surgery. 2018;**22**(1):97

[26] Chen MW, Akinboyo IC, Sue PK, Donohue PK, Ghanem KG, Detrick B, et al. Evaluating congenital syphilis in a reverse sequence testing environment. Perinatol. 2019;**39**(7):956-963

[27] Thorley N, Adebayo M, Smit E, Radcliffe K. The management of isolated positive syphilis enzyme immunoassay results in HIV-negative patients

attending a sexual health clinic. International Journal of STD & AIDS. 2016;**27**(9):798-800

[28] Wang KD, Xu DJ, Su JR. Preferable procedure for the screening of syphilis in clinical laboratories in China. Infectious Diseases (Lond). 2016;**48**(1):26-31

[29] Eldin C, Jaulhac B, Mediannikov O, Arzouni JP, Raoult D. Values of diagnostic tests for the various species of spirochetes. Médecine et Maladies Infectieuses. 2019;**49**(2):102-111

[30] Withers K, Bristow C, Nguyen M, Stafylis C, Giang LM, Klausner JD. A field evaluation of a rapid dual immunoassay for human immunodeficiency virus and syphilis antibodies, Hanoi, Vietnam. International Journal of STD AIDS. 2019;**30**(2):173-180

[31] Caswell RJ, Hathorn E, Manavi K. The significance of isolated reactive treponemal enzyme immunoassay in the diagnosis of early syphilis. Sexually Transmitted Diseases. 2016;**43**(6):365-368. DOI: 10.1097/OLQ.0000000000000446

[32] Huh HJ, Chung JW, Park SY, Chae SL. Comparison of automated treponemal and nontreponemal test algorithms as first-line syphilis screening assays. Annals of Laboratory Medicine. 2016;**36**(1):23-27. DOI: 10.3343/alm.2016.36.1.23

[33] Murai R, Yamada K, Yonezawa H, Yanagihara N, Takahashi S. Evaluation of new algorithm using TPLA as an initial syphilis screening test. Journal of Infection and Chemotherapy. 2019;**25**(1):68-70

[34] Palamar M, Degirmenci C, Sertoz R, Aydemir S, Egrilmez S, Yagci A. Serologic evaluation of cornea donors and microbiologic evaluation of cornea storage Media in an eye Bank from Izmir, Turkey. Experiment in Clinical Transplantation. 2017;**15**(6):685-688

[35] Zheng S, Lin RJ, Chan YH, Ngan CCL. Biological false-positive venereal disease research laboratory test in cerebrospinal fluid in the diagnosis of neurosyphilis - a case-control study. Journal of the European Academy of Dermatology and Venereology. 2018;**32**(3):474-481

[36] Ishihara Y, Okamoto K, Shimosaka H, Ono Y, Kanno Y, Ikeda M, et al. Prevalence and clinical characteristics of patients with biologically false-positive reactions with serological syphilis testing in contemporary practice: 10-year experience at a tertiary academic hospital. Sexually Transmitted Infections. 2021;**97**(6):397-401

[37] Wang W, Fan X, Huang X, Yan J, Luan J. Serologic false-positive reactions for syphilis in children of adenoidal hypertrophy:2 case reports and review of the literature. Acta Clinica Belgica. 2021;**76**(1):70-74

[38] Dunseth CD, Ford BA, Krasowski MD. Traditional versus reverse syphilis algorithms: A comparison at a large academic medical center. Practical Lab Medicine. 2017;**28**(8):52-59

[39] Lin JS, Eder ML, Bean S. Screening for syphilis infection in pregnant women: Updated evidence report and systematic review for the US preventive services task force. Journal of the American Medical Association. 2018;**320**(9):918-925. DOI: 10.1001/jama.2018.7769

[40] De Carolis S, Tabacco S, Rizzo F, Perrone G, Garufi C, Botta A, et al. Association between false-positive TORCH and antiphospholipid antibodies in healthy pregnant women. Lupus. 2018;**27**(5):841-846

[41] Nwosu BO, Eleje GU, Obi-Nwosu AL, Ahiarakwem IF, Akujobi CN, Egwuatu CC, et al. Is routine antenatal venereal disease research laboratory test still justified? Nigerian experience. International Journal of Womens Health. 2015;7:41-46

[42] Ahn SS, Jung SM, Yoo J, Lee SW, Song JJ, Park YB. Clinical characteristics of patients with systemic lupus erythematosus showing a false-positive result of syphilis screening. Rheumatology International. 2019;**39**(11):1859-1866

[43] Dan Gheorghe AC, Hodorogea AS, Georgescu CE, Ciobanu A, Nanea IT, Gheorghe GS. Diagnostic pitfalls in a man with systemic lupus erythematous. European Journal of Case Report and Internal Medicine. 2019;**6**(11):001256

[44] Salado-Rasmussen K, Knudsen A, Krarup HB, Katzenstein TL, Gerstoft J. Undetectable hepatitis C virus RNA during syphilis infection in two HIV/HCV-co-infected patients. Scandinavian Journal of Infectious Diseases. 2014;**46**(9):617-623

[45] Mao CH, Shen M. Peripheral neuropathy caused by cryoglobulinaemia with false-positive serological tests of syphilis. Chinese Medical Journal. 2013;**126**(10):1996

[46] Mbopi-Keou FX, GCM K, Voundi EV, Jenabian MA, Mboumba Bouassa RS, Talla F, et al. Differential influence of race and environment on indeterminate reactivities to non-treponemal and treponemal antigens by immuno-chromatographic dual syphilis rapid test. Pan African Medical Journal. 2019;**33**:90

[47] Augenbraun M, French A, Glesby M, Sanchez-Keeland L, Young M, Greenblatt R, et al. Hepatitis C virus infection and biological false-positive syphilis tests. Sexually Transmitted Infections. 2010 Apr;**86**(2):97-98. DOI: 10.1136/sti.2009.040360

[48] Bright PD, Smith L, Usher J, Donati M, Johnston SL, Gompels MM, et al. False interpretation of diagnostic serology tests for patients treated with pooled human immunoglobulin G infusions: A trap for the unwary. Clinical Medicine (London, England). 2015;**15**(2):125-129. DOI: 10.7861/clinmedicine.15-2-125

[49] Liu F, Liu LL, Guo XJ, Xi Y, Lin LR, Zhang HL, et al. Characterization of the classical biological false-positive reaction in the serological test for syphilis in the modern era. International Immunopharmacology. 2014;**20**(2):331-336

[50] Bopage RI, Vollmer-Conna U, Shand AW, Post JJ. Sex differences in the significance of isolated reactive treponemal chemiluminescence immunoassay results. Sexually Transmitted Infections. 2018;**94**(3):187-191

[51] Mc Gready R, Kang J, Watts I, Tyrosvoutis ME, Torchinsky MB, Htut AM, et al. Audit of antenatal screening for syphilis and HIV in migrant and refugee women on the Thai-Myanmar border: A descriptive study. F1000Res. 2014;**3**:123

[52] Katz AR, Komeya AY, Tomas JE. False-negative syphilis treponemal enzyme immunoassay results in an HIV-infected case-patient. International Journal of STD & AIDS. 2017;**28**(7):735-737

[53] Mmeje O, Chow JM, Davidson L, Shieh J, Schapiro JM, Park IU. Discordant syphilis immunoassays in pregnancy: Perinatal outcomes and implications for clinical management. Clinical Infectious Diseases. 2015;**61**(7):1049-1053

[54] Sönmez C, Demir T, Sezen F, Kılıç S. Investigation of syphilis coinfection and performance of the Architect syphilis Tp ELISA screening test in HIV positive patients. Turkey Journal of Medical Science. 2018;**48**(6):1129-1134. DOI: 10.3906/sag-1802-16

[55] Motlagh MN, Javid CG. Presentation of ocular syphilis in a HIV-positive patient with false-negative serologic screening. Case Report of Infectious Diseases. 2019;**2019**:8191724

[56] Bristow CC, Kojima N, Lee SJ, Leon SR, Ramos LB, Konda KA, et al. HIV and syphilis testing preferences among men who have sex with men and among transgender women in Lima, Peru. PLoS One. 2018;**13**(10): e0206204

[57] Kalou MB, Castro A, Watson A, Jost H, Clay S, Tun Y, et al. Laboratory evaluation of the Chembio dual path platform HIV-syphilis assay. African Journal of Laboratory Medicine. 2016;**5**(1):433

[58] Shakya G, Singh DR, Ojha HC, Ojha CR, Mishra SK, Malla K, et al. Evaluation of SD Bioline HIV/syphilis duo rapid test kits in Nepal. BMC Infectious Diseases. 2016;**16**(1):450. DOI: 10.1186/s12879-016-1694-9

[59] Grégoire Y, Germain M, Delage G. Factors associated with a second deferral among donors eligible for re-entry after a false-positive screening test for syphilis, HCV, HBV and HIV. Vox Sang. 2018;**113**(4):339-344

[60] Zhu WF, Lei SY, Li LJ. Hepatitis C virus infection and biological false-positive syphilis test: A single-center experience. Hepatobiliary & Pancreatic Diseases International. 2011;**10**(4):399-402. DOI: 10.1016/s1499-3872(11)60067-2

[61] Benzaken AS, Bazzo ML, Galban E, Pinto IC, Nogueira CL, Golfetto L, et al. External quality assurance with dried tube specimens (DTS) for point-of-care syphilis and HIV tests: Experience in an indigenous populations screening programme in the Brazilian Amazon. Sexually Transmitted Infections. 2014;**90**(1):14-18

[62] Sandes VS, Silva SGC, Motta IJF, Velarde LGC, de Castilho SR. Evaluation of positive and false-positive results in syphilis screening of blood donors in Rio de Janeiro, Brazil. Transfusion Medicine. 2017;**27**(3):200-206

[63] Sachdev S, Sharma AK, Sethi S, Garg S, Lamba DS, Sharma RR, et al. Comparative evaluation of enzyme-linked immunosorbent assay with rapid plasma reagin for screening of syphilis in blood donors. Asian Journal of Transfusiion Science. 2018;**12**(2):165-168. DOI: 10.4103/ajts.AJTS_126_17

[64] Theodoropoulos N, Jaramillo A, Penugonda S, Wasik C, Brooks K, Ladner DP, et al. Improving syphilis screening in deceased organ donors. Transplantation. 2015;**99**(2):438-443. DOI: 10.1097/TP.0000000000000323

[65] Naesens R, Vermeiren S, Van Schaeren J, Jeurissen A. False positive Lyme serology due to syphilis: Report of 6 cases and review of the literature. Acta Clinica Belgica. 2011;**66**(1):58-59

[66] Toumanios C, Prisco L, Dattwyler RJ, Arnaboldi PM. Linear B cell epitopes derived from the multifunctional surface lipoprotein BBK32 as targets for the serodiagnosis of lyme disease. mSphere. 2019;**4**:3

[67] Park IU, Chow JM, Bolan G, Stanley M, Shieh J, Schapiro JM. Screening for syphilis with the treponemal immunoassay: Analysis

of discordant serology results and implications for clinical management. The Journal of Infectious Diseases. 2011;**204**(9):1297-1304

[68] Hoover KW, Radolf JD. Serodiagnosis of syphilis in the recombinant era: Reversal of fortune. The Journal of Infectious Diseases. 2011;**204**(9):1295-1296

[69] Dassah ET, Adu-Sarkodie Y, Mayaud P. Performance of syphilis sentinel surveillance in the context of endemic treponematoses: experience from Ghana. BMC Infectious Diseases. 2016;**16**(1):745

[70] Gu WM, Yang Y, Wang QZ, Pan BS, Guo W, Wu L, et al. Comparing the performance of traditional non-treponemal tests on syphilis and non-syphilis serum samples. International Journal of STD & AIDS. 2013;**24**(12):919-925

[71] Nah EH, Cho S, Kim S, Cho HI, Chai JY. Comparison of traditional and reverse syphilis screening algorithms in medical health Checkups. Annals of Laboratory Medicine. 2017;**37**(6):511-515. DOI: 10.3343/alm.2017.37.6.511

[72] Rourk AR, Litwin CM. Evaluation of the BioPlex 2200 syphilis total screen (IgG/IgM) with reflex to an automated rapid plasma reagin test. Journal of Clinical Laboratory Analysis. 2019;**33**(5):e22878

[73] Yen-Lieberman B, Daniel J, Means C, Waletzky J, Daly TM. Identification of false-positive syphilis antibody results using a semiquantitative algorithm. Clinical and Vaccine Immunology. 2011;**18**(6):1038-1040

[74] Zhou J, Liang Y, Zhang J, Cui L. The analyzation and clinical evaluation of ECLIA and CMIA in the detection of Treponema pallidum. Medicine (Baltimore). 2017;**96**(24):e7139. DOI: 10.1097/MD.0000000000007139

[75] Shen X, Liu D, Lin Y, Zhu XZ, Lin LR, Tong ML, et al. The characteristics of beta 2-glycoprotein I-dependent anticardiolipin antibody and blood coagulation status in subjects with classical biological false-positive syphilis reactions. International Immunopharmacology. 2018;**62**:132-138

[76] Wang Q, Lei Y, Lu X, Wang G, Du Q, Guo X, et al. Urea-mediated dissociation alleviate the false-positive Treponema pallidum-specific antibodies detected by ELISA. PLoS One. 2019;**14**(3):e0212893

[77] Leamer NK, Jordan NN, Pacha LA, Latif NH, Garges EC, Gaydos JC. Survey of sexually transmitted disease laboratory methods in U.S. Army Laboratories, 2012. Military Medicine. 2017;**182**(3):e1726-e1732. DOI: 10.7205/MILMED-D-16-00248

[78] Li Z, Feng Z, Liu P, Yan C. Screening for antibodies against Treponema pallidum with chemiluminescent microparticle immunoassay: Analysis of discordant serology results and clinical characterization. Annals of Clinical Biochemistry. 2016;**53**(Pt 5):588-592

[79] Adhikari EH, Frame IJ, Hill E, Fatabhoy R, Strickland AL, Cavuoti D, et al. Abbott ARCHITECT syphilis TP chemiluminescentimmunoassayaccurately diagnoses past or current syphilis in pregnancy. American Journal of Perinatology. 2020;**37**(1):112-118

[80] Tao C, Hao X, Xu W, Zhang J, Pan S, Tao Z, et al. Evaluation of the Elecsys syphilis immunoassay for routine screening of serum samples in China. Scientific Reports. 2017;7(1):9559

[81] Li D, An J, Wang T, Tao C, Wang L. Clinical evaluation of fully automated

Elecsys® syphilis assay for the detection of antibodies of Treponema pallidum. Journal of Clinical Laboratory Analysis. 2016;**30**(6):1164-1168

[82] Enders M, Hunjet A, Gleich M, Imdahl R, Mühlbacher A, Schennach H, et al. Performance evaluation of the Elecsys syphilis assay for the detection of total antibodies to Treponema pallidum. Clinical and Vaccine Immunology. 2015 Jan;**22**(1):17-26

[83] Simčič S, Potočnik M. Serological diagnosis of syphilis: A comparison of different diagnostic methods. Acta Dermatovenerol Alp Pannonica Adriat. 2015;**24**(2):17-20

[84] Song X, Tian L, Zou H, Sun H. Analysis of the clinical diagnosis data of four experimental detection methods for pediatric syphilis. Minerva Pediatric. 2019;**71**(2):144-149

[85] Nutten S. Atopic dermatitis: Global epidemiology and risk factors. Annals of Nutrition & Metabolism. 2015;**66** (Suppl. 1):8-16

[86] Silverberg JI. Public health burden and epidemiology of atopic dermatitis. Dermatologic Clinics. 2017;**35**(3):283-289

[87] Khamaganova IV, Novozhilova OL, Vorontsova IV. Epidemiology of atopic dermatitis. The Russian Journal of Dermatology and Venereology. 2017;**16**(4):21-25

[88] Sacotte R, Silverberg JI. Epidemiology of adult atopic dermatitis. Clinical Dermatology. 2018;**36**(5):595-605

[89] Raciborski F, Jahnz-Rozyk K, Kłak A, Sybilski AJ, Grąbczewska AM, Brzozowska M, et al. Epidemiology and direct costs of atopic dermatitis in Poland based on the National Health Fund register (2008-2017). Postepy Dermatology and Alergology. 2019;**36**(6):727-733

[90] Sendrasoa FA, Ranaivo IM, Razanakoto NH, Andrianarison M, Raharolahy O, Ratovonjanahary VT, et al. Epidemiology and associated factors of atopic dermatitis in Malagasy children. Allergy, Asthma and Clinical Immunology. 2020;**16**:4

[91] Halling AS, Bager P, Skov L, Zachariae C, Wohlfahrt J, Melbye M, et al. The interaction between filaggrin mutations and hard domestic water on the risk of early-onset atopic dermatitis. The British Journal of Dermatology. 2020;**183**(2):406-407

[92] Ražnatović Đurović M, Janković J, Ćirković Λ, Sojcvić Timotijević Z, Rašić J, Vitković L, et al. Impact of atopic dermatitis on the quality of life of children and their families. Italian Dermatology Venereology. 2020;**156**(1):29-35

Chapter 5

Treatment of Bacterial Sexually Transmitted Infections in Resource-Limited Settings

Simeon Chijioke Amadi, Chibuzor Peter Oriji, Joseph Okoeguale, Anthony Chukwuemeka Olobuah and Williams Amebeobari Mube

Abstract

Globally, bacterial sexually transmitted infections (STIs) are a major health challenge. It is more challenging in resource-limited settings, where diagnostic capabilities are limited, health insurance is almost nonexistent and medical bills are settled out-of-pocket. In resource-limited settings, most clinicians adopt the syndromic case management approach for effective treatment due to the paucity of resources. The highest levels of multidrug resistant bacterial STIs have been found in resource-limited countries. The reasons are complex and include poor quality of health services, high burden of disease, lack of accessible, accurate, and confirmed diagnostic assays, ineffective regulations, overuse of antibiotics, inappropriate dosing, and lack of knowledge about the risks of microbial resistance. This chapter thus brings to the fore the challenges of treating bacterial sexually transmitted infections in resource-poor settings and the current evidence on the topic for scholars, researchers, and practitioners.

Keywords: treatment, bacterial, sexually transmitted, infections, resource-limited settings

1. Introduction

Sexually transmitted infection (STI) means organisms that lead to infection after sexual intercourse between two persons, while sexually transmitted disease (STD) simply means an obvious clinical disease that resulted from the STI [1]. Doctors and other health workers are the key stakeholders in the prevention and treatment of STIs [1]. The World Health Organization (WHO) estimates that approximately 340 million new cases of the four main curable STIs (gonorrhea, chlamydial infection, syphilis, and trichomoniasis) occur every year, and 75–85% of them in developing countries [2]. STIs impose an enormous burden of morbidity and mortality in developing countries, both directly through their impact on reproductive and child health, and indirectly through their role in facilitating the sexual transmission of

Human Immuno-deficiency Virus (HIV) infection [3]. The high prevalence of STIs has contributed to the disproportionately high HIV incidence and prevalence in most resource-limited settings [3]. The greatest impact is on women and infants [3]. The World Bank has estimated that STIs, excluding HIV, are the second commonest cause of healthy life years lost by women within the age range of 15–44 age in Africa. These bacterial STIs are also responsible for up to 17% of the total disease burden [4].

These underscore the need for appropriate diagnosis and treatment of STI to mitigate the person-to-person transmission and the associated morbidity and mortality associated with the untreated infection acquired sexually [3, 5, 6]. In resource-poor countries, diagnosis based on causative organisms of STIs remains very difficult as a result of the unavailability of laboratory diagnostics that will direct practitioners on the best treatment modality [3]. In the few centers with laboratory support, tests results for the detection of causative organisms for suspected STIs take days/weeks, to be made available to physicians and this makes early definitive/targeted treatment based on etiologic diagnosis difficult/impossible [3, 7].

To solve this problem of lack of etiologic diagnosis and associated difficulty in the treatment of STIs, the WHO brought out the syndromic case management approach in 1984 to guide the practitioners in effective and timely treatment of STIs [8]. This syndromic case management approach remains the approach to STI treatment adopted in many countries of the world, especially developing countries [8]. This syndromic case management approach is based on the identification of consistent groups of symptoms and easily recognizable signs and treatment that will deal with most, or the most serious, organisms responsible for producing the syndrome [9]. Introduction of additional parameters in the syndromic diagnosis of nonviral sexually transmitted infections in low-resource settings and hence improved management has been advocated but is still far-fetched [10].

Consequently, the highest levels of multidrug resistant bacterial STIs have been found in resource-limited countries [11–13]. The reasons are complex and include poor quality of health services, high burden of disease, and lack of accessible, accurate, and confirmed diagnostic assays, ineffective regulations, overuse of antibiotics, inappropriate dosing, and lack of knowledge about the risks of microbial resistance [13]. Not surprisingly, scholarly reviews on syndromic case management, underscored the need for low-cost and accurate Point-of-Care Tests (POCTs) for the identification, first, of *Chlamidia trachomatis* (CT)/*Neisseria gonorrhea* (NG), and, second, of *Mycoplasma genitalium* (MG)/*Trichomonas vaginalis* (TV) and NG/MG resistance/susceptibility testing [14]. Near-patient POCT molecular assays for CT/NG/TV are commercially available, but the cost and other limitations remain prohibitive, especially in resource-constrained settings [7, 15, 16]. These challenges are driving the development of lower-cost solutions [14]. Also, advocacy and subsidization of available diagnostic, treatment, and prevention facilities or measures will immensely reduce the burden of these conditions in the resource-limited settings [14]. This chapter thus brings to the fore the challenges of treating bacterial sexually transmitted infections in resource-poor settings and the current evidence on the topic for scholars, researchers, and practitioners.

2. Treatment of common bacterial infections acquired sexually

There is a paucity of guidelines for the treatment of bacterial sexually transmitted infections in the resource-limited setting. Study of health seeking behavior of patients in developing countries show that a significant number of people with symptomatic STIs seek treatment in the informal or private sector, from traditional healers, unqualified practitioners, street drug vendors, and from pharmacists and unregulated private practitioners, and they will only attend formal public health services (with trained personnel) after alternative treatments have failed [17]. Self-medication is also widely practiced in most resource-limited settings [17–19]. The reasons for these aberrant behavior/practices include but are not limited to the convenience, seeming low cost, flexible payment arrangements, greater accessibility, and the more confidential, less judgmental, and less stigmatizing nature of the services provided by the practitioners in the informal and the largely unregulated private sector [17].

The operational protocol for the treatment of bacterial sexually transmitted infections in formal public health facilities in the resource-limited settings is the "Syndromic Case Management Approach" recommended by the WHO. And so, in this section, the etiologic diagnosis-based treatment guidelines by the Center for Disease Control will be considered first.

Common sexually transmitted bacterial infections include:

2.1 *Klebsiella granulomatis*

This is an intracellular gram-negative bacterium responsible for the granuloma inguinale (donovanosis). Clinically, the disease is characterized as painless, slowly progressive ulcerative lesions on the genitals or perineum without regional lymph adenopathy; subcutaneous granulomas (pseudo buboes) also might occur. A study in Nigeria observed a prevalence of Klebsiella species of 12.3% among women with suspected genital tract infections in a tertiary hospital [20].

For the laboratory testing for Klebsiella, serologic testing is unhelpful. On gram staining, the organism appears as short, plump, and gram-negative bacilli. They are usually surrounded by a capsule and appear as clear space. The organism can be cultured in the laboratory from a specimen from urethral discharge, cervical discharge, vaginal discharge, etc. in infected patients. Klebsiella is micro-aerophilic and can grow in the presence or absence of oxygen. They have no special cultural requirements. Most species can use citrate and glucose as the sole carbon source and so they grow well in most ordinary culture media. But even so, most patients in the resource-limited settings are treated using the syndromic case management approach due to a lack of personnel and facilities and patronage of unskilled caregivers.

The Center for Disease Control (CDC) United States of America recommends oral Azithromycin, 1 g once weekly or 500 mg once a day for up to 3 weeks and until all lesions of Granuloma Inguinale (Donovanosis) have completely healed. Other recommended regimen includes (a) oral Doxycycline 100 mg twice daily for up to 3 weeks and until all lesions of Granuloma Inguinale (Donovanosis) have completely healed. (b) oral Erythromycin 500 mg orally four times/day for up to 3 weeks and until all lesions of Granuloma Inguinale (Donovanosis) have completely healed. (c) oral Trimethoprim-sulfamethoxazole one double-strength (160 mg/800 mg) twice daily for up to 3 weeks and until all lesions of Granuloma Inguinale (Donovanosis) have completely healed [1].

2.2 *Chlamydia trachomatis*

CT is the agent of the most common bacterial STI worldwide, with a significant clinical, economic, and public health impact [21]. This bacterial sexually transmitted infection is responsible for lymphogranuloma venerum (LGV). Some chlamydial infections may occur without clinical symptoms. Individuals with LGV commonly present with tender inguinal or femoral lymph nodes, which are mostly unilateral. Sometimes, an ulcer which is mostly self-limiting may occur at the site of the infection. Often, these lesions would have disappeared by the time the infected individual is seeking care in the hospital. The prevalence of CT in pregnancy in developing countries is between 7 and 31%. In sub-Saharan Africa, the prevalence of CT among high-risk groups in the 1980s was 2–25% while among the low-risk groups in the same period was 2–29% [22–25]. The prevalence of the organism among high-risk groups in the 1990s was 2–13% and among the low-risk group in the same period was 4–18% [22–25]. This high prevalence is occurring in places where we have a paucity of manpower and equipment for the treatment of patients with the resultant morbidity and mortality associated with the disease.

A definitive LGV diagnosis can be made only with LGV-specific molecular testing (e.g., PCR-based genotyping). These tests can differentiate LGV from non-LGV CT in rectal specimens. However, these tests are not widely available, and results are not typically available in a time frame that would influence clinical management. Therefore, diagnosis is based on clinical suspicion, epidemiologic information, and a CT Nucleic acid Amplification Test (NAAT) at the symptomatic anatomic site, along with the exclusion of other etiologies for proctocolitis, inguinal lymphadenopathy, or genital, oral, or rectal ulcers [26, 27]. Genital or oral lesions, rectal specimens, and lymph node specimens (i.e., lesion swab or bubo aspirate) can be tested for CT by NAAT or culture. NAAT is the preferred approach for testing because it can detect both LGV strains and non-LGV CT strains [28]. Therefore, all persons presenting with proctocolitis should be tested for CT with a NAAT performed on the rectal specimen. The facilities and personnel for these services are unavailable to most persons in the resource-limited settings who require these tests. This is due to poverty, ignorance, and poor governance.

For the treatment of CT cervicitis, the CDC recommends oral Doxycycline 100 milligram orally twice daily for 7 days. For individuals who are at risk for gonorrhea or who live in communities where gonorrhea is prevalent, treatment with potent antibiotics for the causative organism—*Neisseria gonorrhea* (NG)—may be considered. Alternatively, a single dose of oral Azithromycin 1 g may be used for the CT infection. The CDC recommended regimen for chlamydial infection among adolescents and adults includes (a) oral Doxycycline 100 mg twice daily for 1 week (b) oral Azithromycin 1 g in a single dose (c) oral Levofloxacin 500 mg once daily for 1 week. The recommended regimen for chlamydial infection during pregnancy includes oral Azithromycin 1 g in a single.

2.3 *Neisseria gonorrhoeae*

In 1879, Albert Neisser first described the gram-negative diplococcus, *NG*, in discharges from urethral and cervical infections [29]. NG affecting the urethra, endocervix, rectum, and pharynx is common and mostly asymptomatic. Up to 50% of female patients who came down with NG infection of the endocervix also develop a simultaneous rectal infection as a result of the contiguous spread of their genital infection [30]. Three days to 2 weeks postexposure, NG infection will appear and symptoms include abnormal vaginal/mucopurulent discharge, bloody discharge, dysuria, dyspareunia, pruritus vulvae, or even perineal pain. Although most times anorectal examination is normal, erythema or ulceration of the anus may be seen on inspection. Untreated gonococcal infection may lead to transient bacteremia, arthritis, or dermatitis. More severe sequelae, such as endocarditis and meningitis, are rare. Penicillinase-producing NG has rendered penicillin G inadequate therapy for infections caused by this organism.

The prevalence of NG in pregnancy in developing countries is between 10 and 20%. In sub-Saharan Africa, the prevalence of NG among high-risk groups in the 1980s was 7–66%, while among the low-risk groups in the same period was 0.3–40% [22–25]. The prevalence of the organism among high-risk groups in the 1990s was 6–31% and among the low-risk group in the same period was 1.6–9% [28–31]. Interestingly, this high prevalence is occurring in places where we have a paucity of manpower and equipment for the treatment of patients with the resultant high morbidity and mortality associated with the disease.

The confirmatory test for NG is by gram stain of directly visualized discharge or by culturing the organism on selective media, for example, Thayer-Martin. Where lubricant is needed during sample collection, water is recommended for use to avoid the reduction in a culture that may be occasioned by the use of antibacterial-containing lubricants. The non-culture techniques for the diagnosis of NG, for example, NAATs are becoming popular [31] but these diagnostic modalities are far-fetched in the resource-limited settings due to lack of equipment and personnel and also because patients patronize untrained personnel.

The CDC recommends the following treatment—Intramuscular Ceftriaxone 500 mg in a single dose for individuals with a total body weight of less than 150 kg. For patients in whom chlamydial infection has not been ruled out, treatment with oral doxycycline 100 mg twice daily for 7 days may be helpful. Patients who weigh ≥150 kg, should receive intramuscular ceftriaxone 1 g ceftriaxone in a single dose. Alternative treatment entails intramuscular Gentamicin 240 mg in a single dose plus oral Azithromycin 2 g in a single dose or oral Cefixime 800 mg in a single dose [1].

2.4 *Treponema pallidum* (TP)

This bacterium (a spirochete) causes the sexually transmitted disease called syphilis. It is among the oldest known infectious diseases. The categorization of the disease into clinical stages is based on the clinical manifestations, especially if left untreated and this categorization guides the patient's treatment and follow-up. Patients with syphilis might seek treatment or be treated on the basis of signs or symptoms (clinical manifestations). The prevalence of syphilis in pregnancy in developing countries is between 2.5 and 17%. In sub-Saharan Africa, the prevalence of TP among high-risk groups in the 1980s was 4–32%, while among the low-risk groups in the same period was 0.01–33% [22–25]. The prevalence of the organism among high-risk groups in the 1990s was 2–29% and among the low-risk group in the same period was 1–29% [22–25]. In the same vein, this high prevalence is occurring in places where we have a paucity of manpower and equipment for testing and etiologic treatment of patients, with the resultant morbidity and mortality associated with the disease.

Primary syphilis: The classical presentation of primary syphilis is a single painless ulcer (chancre) at the infection site within 2–10 weeks postexposure and it can also manifest with atypical, multiple, or painful lesions [32]. The lesion will ulcerate eventually but heals within 2–4 weeks even without treatment [33].

Secondary syphilis: Hematogenous spread of syphilis occurs 4–10 weeks after primary syphilis and leads to secondary syphilis. This may manifest in the form of skin rash, mucocutaneous lesions, and lymphadenopathy. This age is characterized by nonspecific systemic symptoms, such as fever, malaise, arthralgia, weight loss, sore throat, and headache, in addition to a maculopapular rash on the trunk and extremities. Condyloma latum, which are gray or white wart-like spirochete-filled lesions that also appear in secondary syphilis. They appear adjacent to the primary chancre. If left untreated, the syphilitic symptoms will spontaneously resolve after 3–12 weeks. Relapse of symptoms in the first year (early latent syphilis) may be experienced by ¼ of the patients if the condition is left untreated.

Tertiary syphilis: This may manifest in the form of cardiac conditions, gummatous lesions, tabes dorsalis, and general paresis [32].

Latent syphilitic infections are otherwise subclinical infections (without symptoms and signs) and can be detected through serologic assays. Latent syphilitic infections are classified as (a) early latent syphilis—acquired within the preceding year, (b) late latent syphilis, and (c) latent syphilis of unknown duration.

Central Nervous System (CNS) syphilis, TP infection can spread to the CNS. This can happen at any stage of syphilis and result in neurosyphilis. Within the first few months or years of TP infection, CNS clinical symptoms and signs knowns as syphilitic meningitis can be noticed. These features may include cranial nerve abnormalities, meningitis, meningovascular syphilis, cerebrovascular accident, and acute altered mental state. Tabes dorsalis and general paresis are some of the neurologic features that may be noticed in patients with up to 10 to >30 years of TP infection [1].

The involvement of the ocular/visual system or the auditory system is referred to as ocular syphilis and otosyphilis, respectively. These commonly occur at the early stages of the TP infection and can manifest with or without other CNS affectation. They can also occur at any other stage of the disease. Panuveitis is the most common manifestation of ocular syphilis. Other manifestations of ocular syphilis are affectation of the anterior and posterior segment of the eye, including conjunctivitis, anterior uveitis, posterior interstitial keratitis, optic neuropathy, and retinal vasculitis. Patients with ocular syphilis may develop permanent/irreversible blindness. Clinical manifestations of the otosyphilis are tinnitus, vertigo, and sensorineural deafness. Hearing loss can involve one side of the ear or both sides. The hearing loss may also be sudden in onset and progress fast. Otosyphilis may lead to irreversible deafness.

Dark-field examinations and molecular tests for detecting TP directly from lesion exudate or tissue are the definitive methods for diagnosing early syphilis and congenital syphilis [33]. Syphilis is diagnosed by seeing the spirochetes on a dark-field microscopic exam of scrapings from chancres. The next diagnostic method is a demonstration of spirochetes in biopsy specimens stained with Warthin-Starry silver. Alternatively, a direct fluorescent antibody test for TP is performed by some laboratories [33]. Other investigations include the non-treponemal (not specific for treponemal antibodies) serologic tests, such as rapid plasma regain and Venereal Disease Research Laboratory (VDRL), which have a false-negative rate of up to 25%. If the non-treponemal tests return positive, a confirmatory treponemal test such as the fluorescent treponemal antibody absorption test should be conducted on the patient.

The CDC recommended regimen for primary and secondary syphilis among adults includes benzathine penicillin G 2.4 million units intramuscularly in a single dose. The recommended regimen for syphilis among infants and children includes benzathine penicillin G 50,000 units/kg body weight intramuscularly, up to the adult dose of 2.4 million units in a single dose. For patients with penicillin allergy, the regimen of Doxycycline (100 mg orally two times/day for 14 days) [34, 35] or tetracycline (500 mg orally four times/day for 14 days) have been used for years and can be effective [34, 35]. Due to gastrointestinal side effects, Doxycycline may be preferred to tetracycline.

Most patients in developing countries may not be opportune to have diagnostic investigations carried out for their symptoms before treatment due to a lack of hospitals and trained personnel and poverty. They may even experience delayed or absent treatment with the attendant sequelae.

2.5 *Mycoplasma genitalium*

This infection in women may be symptomatic or asymptomatic. In women infected with these bacteria, there have been such findings as cervicitis, pelvic inflammatory disease (PID), preterm delivery, spontaneous abortion, and infertility, with an approximately two-fold increase in the risk for these outcomes in such women [36]. The prevalence of MG in developed countries with higher Human Development Index (HDI) was 1.3–1.6% but the prevalence in developing countries with lower HDI was 3.9–5.2% [37]. The figures show that the prevalence is lower in developed countries compared to developing countries. Despite this obvious trend, the availability of facilities and personnel for testing, treatment, and prevention of these diseases is limited in developing countries.

This organism grows slowly in the culture medium in the laboratory. It can take up to 6 months to culture this organism and this is mostly limited to research for now. The Food and Drug Administration (FDA) in the USA has approved the use of NAAT for detection of the *MG* from urine, urethral, penile meatal, endocervical, and vaginal swab samples. The needed molecular tests for quinolone and macrolide-resistant testing are not available commercially. Men with recurrent nongonococcal urethritis (NGU) should be tested for MG using an FDA-cleared NAAT. If resistance testing is available, it should be performed, and the results used to guide therapy. Women with recurrent cervicitis should be tested for MG, and testing should be considered among women with pelvic inflammatory disease (PID) [1]. Testing should be accompanied by resistance testing, if available. Screening of asymptomatic MG infection among women and men or extragenital testing for MG is not recommended. In clinical practice, if testing is unavailable, MG should be suspected in cases of persistent or recurrent urethritis or cervicitis and considered for PID [1]. The laboratory confirmation of this organism is tedious and also not available for most patients in developing countries for the same reasons already adduced above.

Treatment: Based on CDC recommendations, if the organism is macrolide sensitive: oral Doxycycline 100 mg twice daily for 7 days, followed by oral Azithromycin 1 g initial dose, followed by 500 mg once daily for 3 additional days (2.5 g total). If macrolide-resistant oral Doxycycline 100 mg daily for 7 days followed by oral moxifloxacin 400 mg once daily for 7 days should be administered.

3. Peculiarities of bacterial STI treatment in resource-limited settings

The above treatment recommendations for bacterial sexually transmitted infections are mostly practicable in developed societies. Some health facilities in the resource-limited settings are able to promptly carry out etiologic diagnosis of bacterial STIs and as such the above guidelines may be very beneficial in the management of patients who seek care in such centers. Nevertheless, there is predominantly a paucity of trained personnel, equipment, hospitals, and even access road to go to the existing health facilities in most parts of these resource-limited countries. The functional tertiary and secondary health facilities in most developing countries are situated in a few cities in such countries. The communities are thus left without adequate coverage by skilled personnel. The diagnosis of STIs in such areas is clinical (based on symptoms and signs) and mostly inaccurate due to a lack of trained personnel and equipment. Consequently, the treatment for bacterial STIs is mostly based on WHO syndromic case management. This entails treatment with a combination of broad-spectrum antibiotics without etiologic diagnosis. Usually, a combination of antibiotics from different classes is employed in the treatment of suspected cases of bacterial STIs [20]. These antibiotics are mostly gotten over the counter in these resource-limited settings. Even so, these disease conditions are treated by patent medicine dealers (who do not have conventional training in health and medicine-related matters) and other health personnel who are not trained and/or licensed for drug prescription/patient treatment. These treatments in resource-limited communities are usually inadequate due to inappropriate choice of drugs, under-dosing, and poor compliance to the prescribed drug regimen occasioned by poverty and ignorance. This results in bacterial antibiotic resistance, immediate and long-term avoidable sequelae of the infections, transmission to other sex partners, and endemicity of such infections in the affected communities.

4. Retesting posttreatment to diagnose recurrent infections

Population-based prevention may be improved through the retesting and diagnosis of chlamydia and gonorrhea 3 months after the initial diagnosis [38, 39]. Patients who were diagnosed with chlamydia or gonorrhea need to be retested 3 months after treatment to exclude recurrent infection and confirm treatment success. The fact that there could be a false diagnosis based only on signs and symptoms, further reemphasizes why retesting after the treatment is important. Also, it is recommended that any patient who had a diagnosis and treatment of syphilis need to have follow-up serologic syphilis screening. These recommendations are difficult to implement in resource-limited settings because most patients patronize the nonregulated private sector where services are mostly provided by untrained personnel.

5. Prevention of the STIs in resource-limited settings

In view of the enormous burden of STIs, especially in developing countries, and the paucity of resources for their testing and treatment, prevention is very cost-effective and more reliable in reducing the morbidity and mortality associated with STIs. Firstly, knowing one's STI status will aid one protect oneself and also protect one's sexual partner from the infection and its sequelae. Many STIs can be easily diagnosed and treated; hence, concurrent treatment of sexual partners who have STIs has been found pivotal in the reduction of new cases and recurrence of the disease. Avoidance of multiple sexual partners is also key to the prevention of STIs in the resource-limited settings. Empowerment of the girl child through skills acquisition or formal education is another very important strategy. Use of barrier methods during sex, for example, condoms have been found to not only protect against STIs but also prevent unwanted pregnancies and their sequelae. Individuals who have allergies to latex condoms can resort to the use of synthetic non-latex condoms. Other multipurpose prevention technologies (for the prevention of STIs and pregnancy) are still at the level of research [1].

Pre-exposure prophylaxis and postexposure prophylaxis for STIs have been shown to aid its prevention. Oral Azithromycin 1 g every month has been found to bring down the number of new cases of both NG and CT but did not reduce the number of new cases of HIV [40]. Due to poverty and ignorance, prophylaxis is difficult in resource-limited settings. Most developing societies are male-dominated and women are unable to negotiate sex due to poverty, ignorance, and hunger and so, the use of barrier methods or even keeping one sex partner is difficult. Furthermore, implementation of some of these primary preventive measures in developing countries are difficult due to communal crisis/wars/terrorism (with citizens living in inhumane conditions in internally displaced person camps), poor leadership and lack of facilities to aid individuals adopt these measures. The females in these communities are not only unable to negotiate sex but are forced into sexual activities and have no authority/agency of government to report or run to for protection. And so, to effectively prevent STIs in resource-limited countries, these issues must be addressed, especially with the aid of technologically advanced/developed countries. Unless we all are protected, none of us is protected.

6. Special considerations

6.1 Detection of bacterial sexually transmitted infection in pregnancy

The transmission of infections sexually during the intrauterine or perinatal period is associated with enormous consequences for both the woman and her fetus(es) or the newborn baby(ies) and even her partner. Sexually transmitted infections (STI) are risk factors for a number of adverse pregnancy outcomes, including spontaneous abortion, stillbirth, prematurity, low birth weight (LBW), postpartum endometritis, and various sequelae in surviving neonates. Preterm birth and low birth weight (LBW) are major determinants of infant morbidity and mortality, especially in developing countries, where neonatal intensive care facilities are often unavailable. In a study in Kenya, the incidence of LBW was 7.5%, and the perinatal mortality in LBW babies was 222 per 1000 live births [41]. STIs are believed to be of particular importance in determining pregnancy outcomes in the developing world because the prevalence of infection is so high [42]. During pregnancy, the gravidae and their partners should discuss with the health workers on the STIs and the risks of intrauterine/perinatal transmission to the fetus/neonate. They should also have access to the screening and treatment options available in their locality. In Nigeria and some other resource-limited settings, the only bacterial STI that has a routine screening at the first antenatal visit is syphilis using the VDRL test. Women with positive results from the VDRL test undergo the confirmatory tests (see the section on TP) and receive appropriate treatment as necessary. In many instances, the only available test in the rural and suburban areas of these developing countries is the VDRL or not at all. And so, treatment is given based on the positive VDRL (non-treponemal) test. The treatment may be inadequate based on wrong drug choice or inappropriate dosage of the correct drugs. Many women do not get tested and do not receive treatment for STIs because they receive care from unskilled personnel outside the health center settings.

6.2 Detection of bacterial sexually transmitted infection among adolescents

Adolescents are at an increased risk of STIs. The risk factors for STIs during the adolescent age are as follows: (a) having multiple sex partners, (b) having sequential sex partnerships of limited duration or concurrent partnerships, (c) none compliance to use barrier protection consistently and correctly, (d) low socioeconomic status, and (e) presence of multiple obstacles to health care access [43, 44]. In some developed countries, such as the United States of America, adolescents are allowed by law to seek STD services without the consent of their parents or caregivers. Their health insurance specifies the care needed by the adolescent and such care is provided as necessary [3]. In most developing countries, such as Nigeria, there is no law protecting adolescents with respect to STD services as parents or caregivers must consent before most adolescents can access care in those countries [45]. This is because health insurance is not available to most adolescents and their parents or caregivers pay out of pocket for their health care and there are no laws guiding the adolescents' health care. Obviously, the majority of adolescents who contract STD(s) have to pay out of their pocket to receive care and they do not have the money. The few that have health insurance got it through their parents and the parents must give permission before such adolescents can access care. This compromises the confidentiality needed for the cooperation of adolescents in STI treatment [3]. These now predispose the adolescents to seek care from the alternative unregulated private sector mainly dominated by the herbalists in those resource-limited communities.

6.3 Use of antibiotics during pregnancy

Discoloration of the teeth is one of the dreaded complications of the use of Doxycycline in pregnancy, but the risk is not properly defined. Doxycycline is safe during breastfeeding [25]. Patients with glucose-6-phosphate dehydrogenase deficiency may have neonates who suffer neonatal jaundice/neonatal kernicterus due to sulfonamide use in pregnancy. And so, sulfonamides should be avoided in the third trimester and during breastfeeding [45]. Macrolide regimen (Erythromycin or Azithromycin) is the best suitable regimen of antibiotic treatment for pregnant and lactating women with granuloma inguinale. And so, pregnancy must be ruled out before the use of antibiotics in a sexually active woman of reproductive age. Again, this is not obtainable in most resource-limited settings due to a lack of trained personnel, ignorance, and poverty. In most developing countries, antibiotics can be bought over-the-counter, and sexually active women will usually go to the untrained personnel in the markets to procure antibiotics for treatment without prior doctors' prescription/evaluation.

7. Conclusions

The World Health Organization (WHO) syndromic case management guidelines should be updated to raise the quality of STI management through the integration of laboratory tests. STI screening strategies are needed in the resource-limited settings to address asymptomatic STIs. Point-of-Care Tests (POCTs) that are accurate, rapid, simple, and affordable are urgently needed in resource-constrained settings to support the uptake of etiological diagnosis and treatment. Continued advocacy and support/aid for these countries and their communities will ensure the success of an updated WHO syndromic management guideline and help reduce the burden and adverse effects of STIs.

Acknowledgements

We are grateful to our families, friends, and colleagues, who assisted in no small way in ensuring the completion of this book chapter.

Author details

Simeon Chijioke Amadi[1*], Chibuzor Peter Oriji[2], Joseph Okoeguale[3], Anthony Chukwuemeka Olobuah[4] and Williams Amebeobari Mube[4]

1 Rivers State University, Port Harcourt, Nigeria

2 Department of Obstetrics and Gynaecology, Federal Medical Centre, Yenagoa, Bayelsa State, Nigeria

3 Irrua Specialist Teaching Hospital, Irrua, Nigeria

4 University of Port Harcourt Teaching Hospital, Port Harcourt, Nigeria

*Address all correspondence to: amachijio@yahoo.com

References

[1] Workowski KA, Bachmann LH, Chan PA, Johnston CM, Muzny CA, Park I, et al. Sexually transmitted infections treatment guidelines. CDC MMWR. 2021;**70**(4):1-135

[2] WHO. Global Prevalence and Incidence of Selected Curable Sexually Transmitted Infections: Overviews and Estimates. WHO/HIV_AIDS/2001.02. Geneva: WHO, 2001. [Accessed: September 2, 2022]

[3] Mayaud P, Mabey D. Approaches to the control of sexually transmitted infections in developing countries: Old problems and modern challenges. Sexually Transmitted Infections. 2004;**80**:174-182. DOI: 10.1136/sti.2002.004101

[4] World Bank. World Development Report 1993: Investing in Health. New York: Oxford University Press for the World Bank, New York; 1993

[5] World Health Organization (WHO). Global Health Care Sector Strategy on Sexually Transmitted Infection, 2016-2021. Geneva: WHO; 2016. Available from: http://www.who.int/reproductivehealth/publications/rtis/ghss-stis/en/ [Accessed: August 30, 2022]

[6] Steen R, Wi T, Kamali A, Ndowa F. Control of sexually transmitted infections and prevention of HIV transmission: Mending a fractured paradigm. Bulletin of the World Health Organization. 2009;**87**(11):858-865

[7] Unemo M, Bradshaw CS, Hocking JS, de Vries HJC, Francis SC, Mabey D, et al. Sexually transmitted infections: Challenges ahead. The Lancet Infectious Diseases. 2017;**17**(8):e235-e279

[8] World Health Organization (WHO). Progress Report on the Implementation of the Global Strategy for the Prevention and Control of Sexually Transmitted Infections; 2006-2015. Geneva: WHO; 2015. Available from: http://www.who.int/reproductivehealth/publications/rtis/STI-progress.pdf

[9] World Health Organization (WHO). Sexually Transmitted and Other Reproductive Tract Infections: A Guide to Essential Practice. Geneva: WHO; 2005. Available from: https://www.who.int/reproductivehealth/publications/rtis/9241592656/en/

[10] Sonkar SC, Arora G, Wasnik K, Ali M, Mittal P, Saluja D. Improved management can be achieved by introducing additional parameters in the syndromic diagnosis of nonviral sexually transmitted infections at low-resource settings. American Journal of Obstetrics and Gynecology Global Reports. 2022;**2**(1):100037

[11] Saleh AM, Abdalla HS, Satti AB, Babiker SM, Gasim GI, Adam I. Diagnosis of Trichomonous vaginalis by microscopy, latex agglutination, diamond's media, and PCR in symptomatic women, Khartoum, Sudan. Diagnostic Pathology. 2014;**9**:49

[12] Trabert B. Risk factors for bacterial vaginosis during pregnancy among African-American women. American Journal of Obstetrics and Gynecology. 2008;**197**:2-7

[13] Filho DSC, Diniz CG, DASilva VL. Bacterial vaginosis: Clinical, epidemiologic and microbiological features. HU Revista Juiz. 2010;**36**:223-230

[14] Wi TEC, Ndowa FJ, Ferreyra C, Kelly-Cirino C, Taylor MM, Toskin I, et al. Diagnosing sexually transmitted infections in resource constrained settings: Challenges and ways forward. Journal of the International AIDS Society. 2019;**22**(S6):e25343

[15] Wi T, Lahra M, Ndowa F, Bala M, Dillon J, Ramon-Pardo P, et al. Antimicrobial resistance in *Neisseria gonorrhoeae*: Global surveillance and a call for international collaborative action. PLoS Medicine. 2017;**14**(7):e1002344

[16] Peeling RWW, Mabey D. Point-of-care tests to reduce the burden of sexually transmitted infections. The Lancet Infectious Diseases. 2019;**19**:570-571

[17] Crabbe F, Carsauw H, Buve A, et al. Why do men with urethritis in Cameroon prefer to seek care in the informal health sector? Genitourinary Medicine. 1996;**72**:220-222

[18] Van der Geest S. Self-care and the informal sale of drugs in South Cameroon. Social Science & Medicine. 1987;**25**:293-305

[19] Khamboonruang C, Beyer C, Natpratan C, et al. Human immunodeficiency virus infection and self-treatment for sexually transmitted diseases among northern Thai men. Sexually Transmitted Diseases. 1996;**23**:264-269

[20] Amadi SC, Mkpe A, Awopeju ATO, Iwo-Amah RS, Olobuah AC. Microbial milieu and antibiogram of female genital infections in a tertiary health Facility in Nigeria. Nigerian Medical Journal. 2022;**63**(5):348

[21] World Health Organization (WHO). Report on Global Sexually Transmitted Infection Surveillance. 2015. Available from: https://www.who.int/reproductivehealth/publications/rtis/stis-surveillance-2015/en/. [Accessed: August 30, 2022]

[22] Mayaud P. Infertility in Africa: The role of reproductive tract infections. In: Boerma T, Mgalla Z, editors. Women and Infertility in Africa: A Multidisciplinary Perspective with Special Reference to Tanzania. Amsterdam: Royal Tropical Institute, KIT Press; 2001

[23] Wasserheit JN, Holmes KK. Reproductive tract infections: Challenges for international health policy, programs, and research. In: Germain A, Holmes KK, Piot P, Wasserheit JN, editors. Reproductive Tract Infections: Global Impact and Priorities for women's Reproductive Health. For IWHC. New York: Plenum Press; 1992. pp. 7-33

[24] Mindel A, Dallabetta G, Gerbase A, Holmes KK. Syndromic approach to STD management. Sexually Transmitted Infections. 1998;**74**(Suppl. (I)):S1-S78

[25] Gerbase AC, Rowley JT, Mertens TE. Global epidemiology of sexually transmitted diseases. Lancet. 1998;**351**(Suppl. III):SIII2-SIII4

[26] Ilyas S, Richmond D, Burns G, et al. Orolabial lymphogranuloma venereum, Michigan, USA. Emerging Infectious Diseases. 2019;**25**:2112-2114. DOI: 10.3201/eid2511.190819

[27] Kersh EN, Pillay A, de Voux A, Chen C. Laboratory processes for confirmation of lymphogranuloma venereum infection during a 2015 investigation of a cluster of cases in the United States. Sexually Transmitted Diseases. 2017;**44**:691-694. DOI: 10.1097/OLQ.0000000000000667

[28] Centers for Disease Control and Prevention. Recommendations for

the laboratory-based detection of Chlamydia trachomatis and Neisseria gonorrhoeae--2014. MMWR Recomm Rep. 14 Mar 2014;**63**(RR-02):1-19. PMID: 24622331; PMCID: PMC4047970

[29] Sullivan EA, Abel M, Tabrizi S, et al. Prevalence of sexually transmitted infections among antenatal women in Vanuatu, 1999-2000. Sexually Transmitted Diseases. 2003;**30**:362-366

[30] Fonck K, Kidula N, Jaoko W, et al. Validity of the vaginal discharge algorithm among pregnant women and non-pregnant women in Nairobi, Kenya. Sexually Transmitted Infections. 2000;**76**:33-38

[31] Gray H, Wabwire-Mangen F, Kigozi G, et al. Randomized trial of presumptive sexually transmitted disease therapy during pregnancy in Rakai, Uganda. American Journal of Obstetrics and Gynecology. 2001;**185**:1209-1217

[32] Towns JM, Leslie DE, Denham I, Azzato F, Fairley CK, Chen M. Painful and multiple anogenital lesions are common in men with *Treponema pallidum* PCR-positive primary syphilis without herpes simplex virus coinfection: A cross-sectional clinic-based study. Sexually Transmitted Infections. 2016;**92**:110-115

[33] Theel ES, Katz SS, Pillay A. Molecular and direct detection tests for *Treponema pallidum* subspecies *pallidum*: A review of the literature, 1964-2017. Clinical Infectious Diseases. 2020;**71**(Suppl. 1):S4-S12. DOI: 10.1093/cid/ciaa176

[34] Ghanem KG, Erbelding EJ, Cheng WW, Rompalo AM. Doxycycline compared with benzathine penicillin for the treatment of early syphilis. Clinical Infectious Diseases. 2006;**42**:e45-e49

[35] Wong T, Singh AE, De P. Primary syphilis: Serological treatment response to doxycycline/tetracycline versus benzathine penicillin. The American Journal of Medicine. 2008;**121**:903-908

[36] Lis R, Rowhani-Rahbar A, Manhart LE. *Mycoplasma genitalium* infection and female reproductive tract disease: A meta-analysis. Clinical Infectious Diseases. 2015;**61**:418-426

[37] Baumann L, Cina M, Egli-Gany D, Goutaki M, Halbeisen FS, Lohrer G. Prevalence of mycoplasma genitalium in different population groups: Systematic review and meta-analysis. Sexually Transmitted Infections. 2018;**94**:254-261

[38] Turner AN, Feldblum PJ, Hoke TH. Baseline infection with a sexually transmitted disease is highly predictive of reinfection during follow-up in Malagasy sex workers. Sexually Transmitted Diseases. 2010;**37**:559-562

[39] Peterman TA, Tian LH, Metcalf CA, et al. High incidence of new sexually transmitted infections in the year following a sexually transmitted infection: A case for rescreening. Annals of Internal Medicine. 2006;**145**:564-572

[40] Kaul R, Kimani J, Nagelkerke NJ, et al. Monthly antibiotic chemoprophylaxis and incidence of sexually transmitted infections and HIV-1 infection in Kenyan sex workers: A randomized controlled trial. JAMA. 2004;**291**:2555-2562

[41] Mati J, Aggarwal V, Lucas S, et al. The Nairobi birth survey. 1. The study design, the population and outline results. Journal of Obstetrics & Gynaecology of Eastern and Central Africa. 1982;**1**:132-139

[42] World Health Organization. Global Prevalence and Incidence of Selected Curable Sexually Transmitted Infections:

Overview and Estimates. Geneva: WHO; 2001

[43] CDC. Sexually Transmitted Disease Surveillance 2019 [Internet]. Atlanta GA: US Department of Health and Human Services, CDC; 2021. Available from: https://www.cdc.gov/std/statistics/2019/default.htm

[44] Leichliter JS, Dittus PJ, Copen CE, Aral SO. Trends in factors indicating increased risk for STI among key subpopulations in the United States, 2002-2015. Sexually Transmitted Infections. 2020;**96**:121-123. DOI: 10.1136/sextrans-2019-054045

[45] Briggs GC. Drugs in Pregnancy and Lactation: A Reference Guide to Fetal and Neonatal Risk. 11th ed. Philadelphia, PA: Wolters Kluwer; 2017

Chapter 6

Neisseria gonorrhoeae Ketol-Acid Reductoisomerase Is a Potential Therapeutic Target

Emna Rigane and Susu M. Zughaier

Abstract

The host-adapted human pathogen *Neisseria gonorrhoeae* is the causative agent of sexually transmitted infection gonorrhea. The increased emergence of gonorrhea infections worldwide, associated with the surging resistance to antimicrobial treatments is alarming. Antimicrobial resistance (AMR) is a global threat to human health and occur through various molecular mechanisms. This research aims to identify molecular therapeutic targets in *N. gonorhoeae* as a potential antibiotic adjuvant. This work is focused on ketol acid reductor-isomerase enzyme (KARI), an enzyme involved in the branched-chain amino acids biosynthesis. A BLASTp analysis revealed that KARI enzyme is highly conserved in *N. gonorrhoeae* strains and present in important bacterial pathogens including ESKAPE. Sequence alignment of different KARI proteins from various human bacterial pathogens and gut microbiota demonstrate that residues forming the active site and cofactors binding sites are conserved among all tested KARIs. A 3D homology-based model for gonococcal KARI was generated using Swiss model server and the KARI template from *S. aureus*. The generated 3D KARI model shows that this enzyme adapts a different conformation upon binding of cofactors, allowing the substrate binding and catalysis, while the active site adapts a closed state.

Keywords: *N. Gonorhoeae*, KARI- enzyme, therapeutic target, ESKAPE pathogens, antimicrobial resistance

1. Introduction

Sexually transmitted infections (STIs) are a major public health problem worldwide, affecting the quality of life and causing serious morbidity and mortality. Indeed, *Neisseria gonorrhoeae* (also known as the gonococcus) is the etiological agent of gonorrhea, the second most frequently reported sexually transmitted infection (STI) in the world [1] after *Chlamydia trachomatis*. This bacterium is a Gram-negative diplococcus that can affect both men and women, causing the infection of the urogenital, rectal, and pharyngeal sites [2].

Clinically, gonorrhea may be asymptomatic in many cases. However, clinical manifestations in men include dysuria, pain in the testicles, and purulent urethral discharge with mucoid secretion from the penis. For women, painful urination, itching, or vaginal discharge might be noticed. Gonorrhea can also infect the rectum inducing pain with bowel movements, constipation or rectal discharge [2], and other sites such as the oropharyngeal mucosa, ocular, and anal mucosa.

Gonococcal infection can induce serious complications, ranging from salpingitis and epididymitis to pelvic inflammatory disease, ectopic pregnancy, and infertility. Gonococcal infection during pregnancy can cause various complications since the infection could be transmitted to newborns via vaginal delivery, which may cause neonatal ophthalmia. Untreated *N. gonorrhoeae*, and other STIs, were shown to facilitate the transmission and acquisition of the human immunodeficiency virus [2]. The control of gonorrhea relies on prevention, appropriate diagnostics, and effective antimicrobial treatment [3].

1.1 Pathogenesis of *N. gonorrhoeae*

In order to establish infection, *N. gonorrhea* first establishes colonization of the mucosal epithelium by adherence and attachment to various epithelial surfaces. This is the first step in pathogenesis, which is mediated by specific bacterial surface structures, including pili type IV (retraction) and opacity (Opa) proteins. The pili type IV retraction brings the gonococci to the cell surface and enable interactions with other surface structures [4].

The next step following adherence is replication of *N. gonorrhoeae,* colonies formation and possibly biofilms. An invasion and transcytosis occur with possible competition with the resident microbiota. During these initial stages in gonococcal infection, *N. gonorrhoeae* produces or sheds lipopolysaccharides, fragments of peptidoglycan, and outer membrane vesicles. The latter could activate Toll-like receptors signaling in epithelial cells, dendritic cells, and macrophages, leading to the release of cytokines and chemokines and then activation of the inflammatory transcription factor. These innate immune signaling pathways allow the recruitment a large number of polymorphonuclear leukocytes to the site of infection where they interact with and phagocytose *N. gonorrhoeae*. The gonococcal colonization could result in symptomatic or asymptomatic infection. In case of sufficient neutrophil influx into the site of infection, a symptomatic infection may occur [4].

Furthermore, *N. gonorrhoeae* avoids clearance by the host immune system in a process known as antigenic variation, due to pili type IV. During this process, gonorrhea alters its cell surface antigens by replacing portions of the expressed pilin gene (*pilE*) with segments of the silent pilin gene (*pilS*) through homologous recombination [5]. *N. gonorrhoeae* could also modulate the host iron innate immune defenses to survive intracellularly under limited bioavailability of iron. This bacterium can survive in association with monocytes and macrophages. Gonococcal stimulation of macrophages influences the pro-inflammatory response, leading to damage during natural infection [6].

1.2 Signs and symptoms

The gonorrhea infection is asymptomatic in more than 70% of infections, especially among females [7]. However, some symptoms may occur such as dysuria (frequent/painful urination), vaginal discharge (watery, creamy, or slightly green), itching/burning in the vaginal area, and bleeding from the vagina between periods.

Affected women can also have purulent or mucopurulent endocervical, commonly referred to as mucopurulent cervicitis [8].

Infection in the uterus and the fallopian tubes were also reported, leading to a painful infection of the pelvis, known as pelvic inflammatory disease (PID). As a result, a tubal pregnancy will occur and can lead to miscarriage and even death of the mother [9]. Pelvic infection causes fever, pain during intercourse, and pelvic pain. In case of severe infection, a tubo-ovarian abscess can be formed and can be fatal, requiring major surgery [9]. Other symptoms of gonorrhea in women include also lower stomach aches. Gonorrhea infection in men can affect the genital tract, leading to burning and painful urination, a pus-like discharge from the tip of the penis (white, green, or yellow), and pain or swelling in one of the testicle (less common) [10]. A throat infection and pain can also occur after a gonorrhea infection in men [11]. Gonorrhea can also affect the rectum, causing pain with bowel movements, rectal discharge, constipation, soreness, itching, bleeding, and discharge. The presence of gonorrhea is also considered as a co-factor in human immunodeficiency virus (HIV) transmission [12].

Accordingly, diagnosis requires appropriate laboratory tests for confirmation, case finding, and antimicrobial testing. Gonorrhea diagnosis is performed through the detection of the bacterium or its genetic material in the human body (genital or extragenital specimens) using culture test, microscopy, or nucleic acids amplification tests. Antimicrobial resistance (AMR) testing of gonococcal isolates should be a crucial part of laboratory diagnosis [13].

1.3 Diagnosis of gonorrhea

In case of symptomatic men infection with urethral discharge, diagnosis can be observed by microscopy, identifying gonococci as intracellular Gram-negative diplococci in polymorphonuclear leukocytes (magnification, ×1000). This cheap method is highly sensitive and specific, can provide rapid results and enables a complete AMR testing. Nonetheless, this method depends on the presence of discharge or secretions, and requires good optimization of many parameters, such as sample collection, storage and transport, culture methodology, as gonococci are fastidious i.e. highly sensitive to external environmental factors [13].

However, in the case of cervical, rectal, or pharyngeal gonorrhea, microscopy is not recommended, especially for asymptomatic patients; in fact that negative results do not exclude the presence of infection due to the low sensitivity of this method. Generally, the microscopy method does not provide any data on antimicrobial sensitivity. In settings with more resources, nucleic acids amplification tests could replace culture for the detection of gonococci. This method allows the detection of nonviable bacterium, with a higher sensitivity than other diagnostic methods, especially for rectal and pharyngeal samples. This method is also rapid, could be automated, and enable simultaneous detection of several pathogens, but it does not inform about antimicrobial resistance profile testing [13].

1.4 Treatment of *gonorrhea*

The empiric treatment of gonococcal infection recommended by the WHO was dual therapy (injectable ceftriaxone and azithromycin). However, some countries have transitioned to ceftriaxone monotherapy (increasing dose from 250 to 500 mg intramuscular injection). This is due to the increasing emergence of azithromycin resistance and the treatment failure of dual therapy as it was reported in 2014 and 2018 in the United Kingdom (UK). This therapeutic strategy has been adapted by other countries, such as the UK, China, and Japan.

Pharyngeal infections are one of the typical treatment failure consequences as they are an important site of infection. Although they are predominantly asymptomatic. This is a warning that the era of untreatable gonorrhea is near, but new drugs that specifically target antibiotic-resistant *N. gonorrhoeae* is under current investigation. Currently, several promising agents are on the horizon for *N. gonorrhoeae*, including new antibiotics. Some new antibiotics target the GyrB subunit in DNA gyrase, such as zoliflodacin, and other target the topoisomerase IV, like the gepotidacin [14].

1.5 *Neisseria gonorrhoeae* antimicrobial resistance and epidemiology

N. gonorrhoeae has a great ability to develop resistance mechanism to available first-line antibiotics, such as penicillin, fluoroquinolones, and tetracyclines, increasing the burden of multidrug-resistant *N. gonorrhoeae* [15]. The study of the evolution of antimicrobial resistance (AMR) shows that the resistance of *N. gonorrhoeae* has been driven by the widespread use and misuse of antibiotics, in view of the natural absence of AMR elements in this bacterium [2]. With the introduction of each new antibiotic, resistance soon followed: penicillins (1943, resistance developed since 1989), fluoroquinolones (the 1980s, no longer recommended in 2007), tetracyclines (1962, high-level resistance noted in 1985), sulfonamides (1930s, up to 90% resistance reported in 1940), spectinomycin (1961, emergence of resistance in 1987), and azithromycin (1983, no longer recommended in 2007), cefixime (1983, clinical failures in Japan in 2010), and ceftriaxone (1980, first high-level resistance strain reported in 2009). Ceftriaxone is presently the last remaining empiric treatment option, highlighting the urgent need for research and development of new antibiotics and change in treatment regimens [2].

Indeed, the treatment failure, slow update of treatment guidelines in most countries, and the particular ability of the gonococci to develop and retain AMR make the global problem of gonococcal AMR worst in the foreseeable future. Consequently, severe complications of gonorrhea will emerge as a silent epidemic [13]. In fact, the WHO lists *N. gonorrhoeae* as a "priority pathogen", and reported over 78 million cases each year, with uncontrolled transmission and limited treatment options, untreatable gonorrhea will increase the incidence and complications from infections, like the infertility in women. Accordingly, the WHO established the Gonococcal Antimicrobial Surveillance Program (GASP) in 1992, to encourage countries to collect and report their AMR data for at least one antibiotic, in order to develop their own gonococcal AMR surveillance programs. Hence, the implementation of optimal surveillance programs is of utmost importance [2].

1.6 Antimicrobial resistance mechanisms in *N. gonorrhoeae*

N. gonorrhoeae is capable to damage its own genetic material because it is naturally competent for transformation during its life cycle and through different types of mutations [13]. This allows bacteria to survive and rapidly adapt to various environments (different sites in the human host). Gonococci develop all mechanisms of AMR to all antimicrobials used or recommended for treatment, e.g., (i) decreasing of the influx of antimicrobial and increasing of their efflux, (ii) modification of targets and reduction of affinity for antimicrobials, and (iii) enzymatic modification or destruction of antimicrobials [13]. As an example, gonococcal resistance to penicillin and tetracycline is due to the mutation of *blaTEM* gene and the *tetM* [16], respectively, which are plasmid-borne and can be easily transferred.

AMR genetic determinants are chromosomally transcribed where some can provide high resistance levels *in vitro* and *in vivo* leading to treatment failure. The acquisition of a single AMR determinant could confer only a cumulative increase in AMR compared to the cumulative effect of certain AMR determinants. The interaction between them may result in a significant increase in AMR levels. For example, the development of several chromosomally inserted determinants results in the resistance of *N. gonorrhoeae* to penicillin.

This looming health threat has restimulated interest in the development of new antimicrobial therapies. Active efforts are being made by several pharmaceutical majors to identify the drug targets and develop new drugs to treat such diseases effectively [17]. These targets should be present in microbes and plants, but not in humans.

Based on previous studies, the branched-chain amino acid (BCAA) pathway has been considered an attractive target for antimicrobial drug discovery as a result of comparative pathway analysis between host and pathogen [17]. First, it has been shown that all enzymes in the pathway are essential for the growth of bacteria in culture. Second, this pathway is present only in bacteria, plants, and fungi but not in animals and humans. Hence, inhibitors that target these enzymes are likely to be nontoxic to humans [18].

The BCAA pathway I is responsible for the synthesis of Leucine, valine, and isoleucine. However, this metabolic pathway is absent in humans and other animals, making them unable to synthesizee their own BCAAs and rely on obtaining these essential nutrients from their diet. Consequently, BCAA enzyme inhibitors are likely to be effective drugs, while not exerting any toxic effects in humans [1]. Ketol-acid reductor-isomerase (KARI) is the second enzyme in the branched-chain amino acid (BCAA) biosynthesis, which regulates many physiological activities in a variety of organisms from bacteria to fungi and plants. The conservation in fungi but absence in mammals of the BCAA biosynthetic pathway makes it the target for herbicides, fungicides, and antimicrobial compounds [19]. KARI catalyzes the conversion of 2-acetolactate and 2-aceto-2-hydroxybutyrate to 2,3-dihydroxyisoverate and 2,3-dihydroxy-3-methyl valerate, respectively. ILVC is a bifunctional enzyme that catalyzes two quite different reactions, but occurs at a common active site, acting both as an isomerase and as a reductase [19].

Previous studies showed the efficiency of some KARI inhibitors against *S. aureus*, *M. tubercul*osis with an inhibitory effect on bacterial growth leading to the killing of bacteria [1, 20]. By assessing the presence of the KARI enzyme in pathogens and understanding its structure and draggability, the design of novel antimicrobials to circumvent the resistance problems can be undertaken more rationally.

This review focuses on looking for the presence of the KARI enzyme among pathogens, bacteria, and fungi, the study of its expression and production during the host infection, and its common druggable site and susceptibility to previously recommended enzyme inhibitors.

2. Material and methods

2.1 Phylogenetic analysis

BLAST searches were carried out to identify different procaryotic ortholog of the *N. gonorrhoeae* (GenBank accession number EEZ44675.1) KARI protein which is conserved in *Neisseria* (https://www.ncbi.nlm.nih.gov/ipg/EEZ44675.1). KARI sequences were aligned using ClustalW [21], and then a neighbor-joining tree was generated using MEGA software [22]. KARI sequences from *Escherichia coli* K12 (AKD89606.1) *Enterococcus faecium* (KXH23108), *Staphylococcus aureus* (MBU4945389.1), *Klebsiella pneumoniae* (MBC4258974.1), *Actinobacter baumanii* (EHU1490884.1), *Pseudomonas aeruginosa* (EJY59157.1), were used for phylogenetic analysis.

2.2 Sequence alignments and phylogenetic analysis

Multiple-sequence alignments were performed using the Clustal W webserver. The evolutionary relationship of *N. gonorrhoeae* to other pathogenic strains producing similar ketol-acid reductor-isomerase enzymes was examined using a phylogenetic analysis of the full-length KARI sequences with the MEGA software (version 11.0.10).

2.3 Homology modeling

The structural model of KARI was obtained from NCBI database http://www.blast.ncbi.nlm.nih.gov. Ketol acid reductor-isomerase (KARI) enzyme of *N. gonorrhoeae* was subjected for homology modeling using the Swiss model. The structural homolog, which was used as a template for this model, is ketol acid reducto-isomerase enzyme from *S. aureus (Sa* KARI*)* with PDB identifier 5w3k. The sequence similarity between the template and the model is about 33%. The KARI model and the template (5w3k) were superimposed using the PYMOL software (version 2.4.1) [23].

3. Results and discussion

3.1 Phylogenetic analysis of KARI from pathogens

According to the results of the BLAST search with the sequence of KARI protein from *Neisseria gonorrhoeae* FA19 (*Ng* KARI), KARI sequences for human pathogens were obtained. A phylogenetic analysis of the amino acid sequence with reported pathogens was conducted. As shown in the result, *Ng* KARI is closely related to the KARI from the ESKAPE pathogens. All of them are clustered in respective clades (**Figure 1a**).

The sequence alignment of KARI protein from other human pathogens is reported in **Figure 1b**. All tested pathogens share a common ancestor. However, KARI from *S. pneumonia*, *N. meningitidis*, *S. enterica*, *M. tuberculosis*, *B. cereus* and *B. anthracis* belong to a different clade than the other pathogens (*Shigella dysenteriae*, *Shigella flexneri*, *Shigella sonnei*, *Yersinia pseudotuberculosis*, *Yersinia enterocoliticia*, and *Francisella pneumoniae*).

The presence of KARI was also assessed in various members of the gut microbiota, to understand if the latter will be inhibited by KARI inhibitors (**Figure 2**). KARI from *P. dentalis* and *B. fragilis* belong to the same clade, different from the other Gut bacteria (*F. nucleatum*, *B. bifidum*, *Lactobacillus* sp., and *A. muciniphila*).

3.2 KARI sequence alignment

The alignment of KARI enzyme was carried out using BLAST and Clustal W. Multiple-sequence alignment of *Ng* KARI and KARIs from human pathogens,

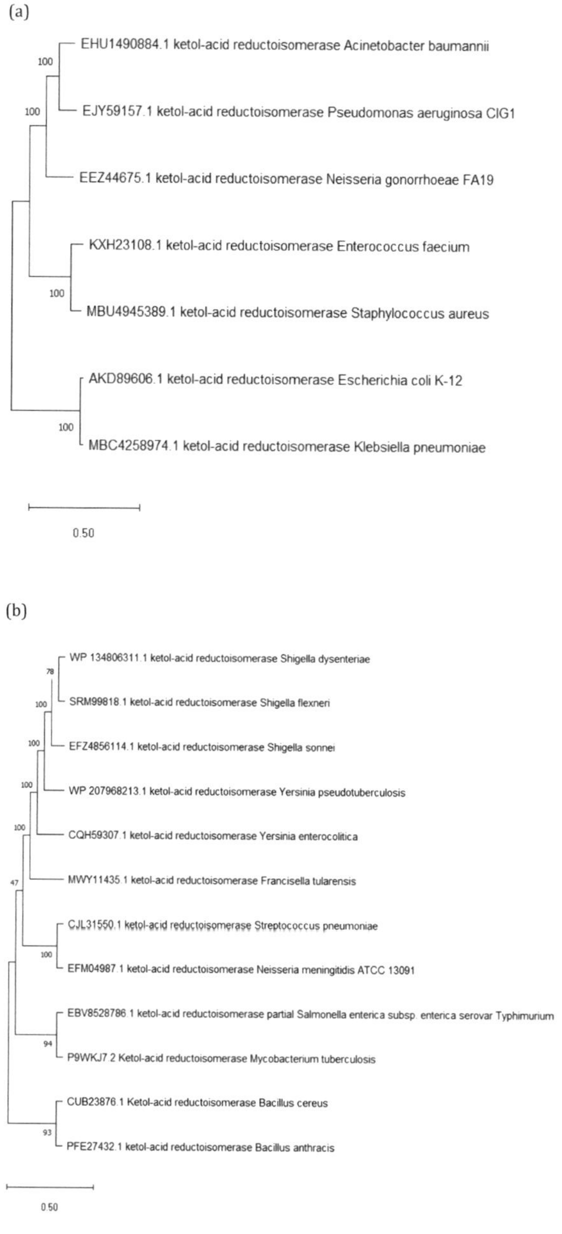

Figure 1.
Phylogenetic tree based on KARI sequence between N. gonorrhoeae and ESKAPE pathogens (a) and other human pathogens (b). Accession numbers are as follows: (a) A. baumannii (EHU1490884), P. aeruginosa CIG1 (EJY 59157), E. faecium (KXH23108), S. aureus (MBU4945389), E. coli K12 (AKD89606), and K. pneumoniae (MBC4258974). (b) S. dysenteriae (WP 134806311.1), S. flexneri (SRM99818.1), S. sonnei (SRM99818.1), Y. pseudotuberculosis (WP 207968213), Y. enterocolitica (CQH59307.1), F. tularensis (MWY11435.1), S. pneumoniae (CJL31550.1), N. meningitidis ATCC 13091 (EFM04987.1), S. enterica (EBV8528786.1), M. tuberculosis (9WKJ7.2), B. cereus (CUB23876.1), and B. anthracis (PFE27432.1).

revealed that residues constituting NADP(H) and Mg^{2+} binding sites are well conserved, while the overall length of each KARI is different. The tested bacteria share different residues, especially in the active pocket, and cofactors binding sites. Indeed, different KARIs have almost identical active site structures.

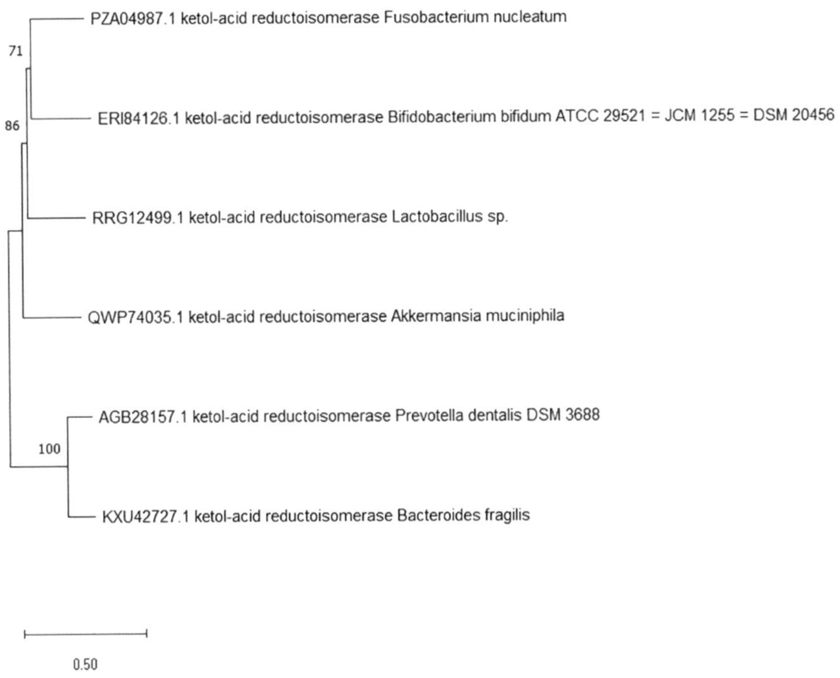

Figure 2.
Phylogenetic tree based on KARI sequence between N. gonorrhoeae and some members of the gut microbiota. Accession numbers are as follows: (a) F. nucleatum (PZA04987.1), B. bifidum (ERI84126), Lactobacillus (RRG12499), A. muciniphila (QWP74035), P. dentalis (AGB28157), and B. fragilis (KXU42727). The tree was constructed using neighbor-joining analysis based on KARI protein sequences. The scale bar represents 0.5 substitutions per nucleotide position.

Analysis of residues contacting NADP(H) and Mg^{2+} identified five amino acid residues, in *Sa* KARI, as contacting ones: Arg-47, Asp-81, Ser-51, Asp-189, and Glu-193 (**Figure 3b**). KARIs harbor a GxGxxG motif, which is part of the nucleotide-binding site by phosphate-bridging interaction (**Figure 3c**), and Mg^{2+} is required for NADP(H) binding. The study of residue mutations' effect on NADPH binding to the KARI's structure show that residues A71, R76, and S78 are in the loop connecting the β2 sheet and the αB helix, referred to as the β2αB loop. R76, and S78 establish direct contact with the 2′-phosphate of NADPH. Sequence alignment of KARI show a variable length of the β2αB loop among tested bacteria (**Figure 4**). This loop is crucial for the cofactor specificity [24].

Upon the binding of cofactors, NADP(H) and Mg^{2+}, the N-terminal domain of KARI undergoes large local conformational changes, only in the NADP(H) binding site. Four Mg^{2+}-binding residues are also identified (D190, E194, E226, and E230) [19]. The side chains of these residues rotate upon metal ion binding. Previously, the mutation of R47 and D81 induce rotameric changes in other bulky residues (His-31, Lys-52, Phe-54, and His-135), resulting in the NADP(H) binding pocket broadening, and then a weak binding to the structure [25].

Other conserved residues are identified. According to available KARI's structure analysis, these amino acids interact with inhibitors. Notably, KARI binds different ligands other than metal ions and NADP(H), such as IpOHA, cyclopropane-1, 1 dicarboxylic acid (CPD) and 2-(dimethyl phosphoryl)-2-hydroxyacetic acid

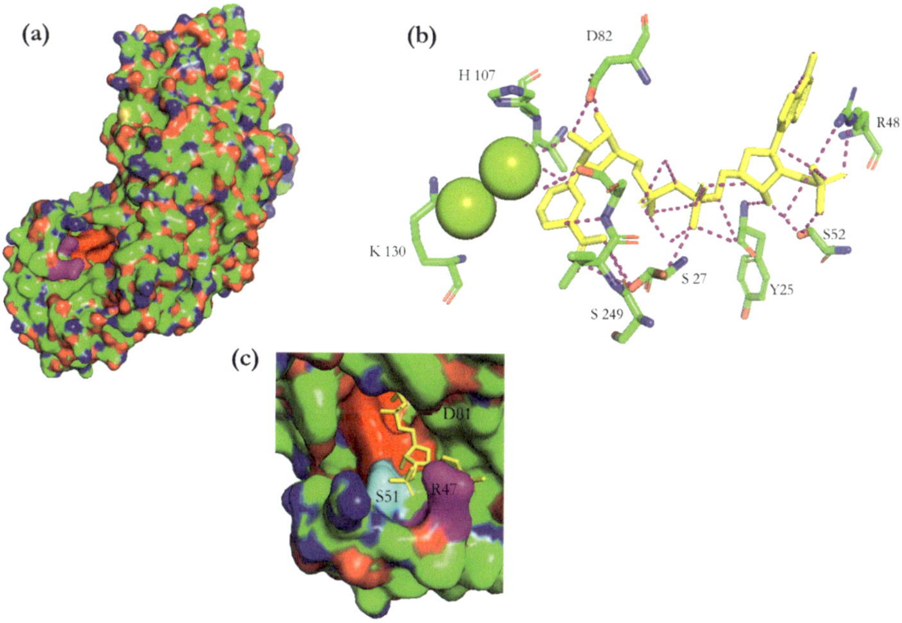

Figure 3.
Surface representation of the crystal structure of KARI from Staphylococcus aureus (Sa KARI) (PDBID: 5w3k) (Sa KARI), the NADP(H) binding site is shown as a red cavity. (b) Stereo view of the binding mode of NADP(H). NADP(H) is shown as yellow sticks, and metals are shown as green spheres. Polar contacts with residues within 5 of the NADPH are shown in magenta in dashed lines (c) surface representation of the NADP(H) binding site pocket of Sa KARI. NADP(H) is shown as yellow sticks.

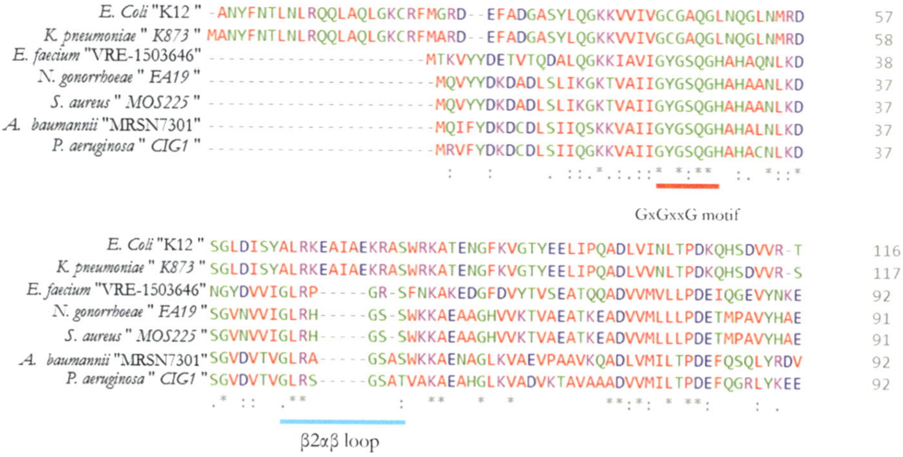

Figure 4.
Multiple alignments of KARI partial sequence from members of the ESKAPE pathogens groups. Clustal W was used to align KARI sequences from six members of the ESKAPE (Escherichia coli strain K12, Staphylococcus aureus strain MOS225, Klebsiella pneumoniae strain K783, Acinobacter baumannii strain MRSN7301, Pseudomonas aeruginosa strain CIG1, and Entercoccus faecium strain VRE-1503646) against the orthologue from N. gonorrhoeae. The alignments were used to identify regions possessing the greatest similarities. The conservation of residues is indicated above the alignments as follows: asterisk, complete identity; colon, conservation of a strong group; period, conservation of a weak group. GxGxxG motif is shown in red line, while β2αB loop is shown in blue line.

Inhibitor	Ligands	PDBID	Reference
CPD	E230	5W3K	[12]
	S251		
	NDP		
	Me^{2+} ions		
IpOHA	D188,	4YPO	[12]
	E192		
	E224		
	E228		
	Mg^{2+} ions		
Tartaric acid	D190	4TSK	[13]
	E194		
	C199		
	G230		
	S251		
	NDP		
Cyclopentylamino(oxo) acetic acid	E193	6C5N	
	D189		
	E229		
	S250		
	Mg^{2+} ions		

Table 1.
Summarization of ligands residues for KARI's inhibitors.

(Hoe704). These compounds are the most extensively characterized KARI inhibitors investigated to date. They are transition state analogs. Residues involved in these inhibitors binding are conserved among bacteria, as described in **Table 1**. These inhibitors could be tested with KARI from *N. gonorrhoeae*, to assess its effect on bacterial growth rate, its viability, and antimicrobial resistance.

In the presence of Mg^{2+} ions, the active site of KARI becomes open and accessible to solvent, while the NADP(H) binding reduces the space between the domains, and the active site adopt a closed conformation. Hence, the active site changes its surface structure to become appropriate for substrate binding. The open-close transition state has been thought to facilitate substrate binding and catalysis. This feature provides then possibilities for the development of inhibitors able to bind to both of structural conformations of KARI (i.e. ± NADPH) [6].

3.3 KARI modeling

The modeling of KARI enzyme from *N. gonorrhoeae* was carried out using the Swiss-model webserver, using as a template the KARI enzyme from *Staphylococcus aureus* (PDBID 5w3k). As shown in **Figure 5**, the KARI model shows high similarity in the active pocket (AFAHGFNIH) and N-terminal and C-terminal domains. A

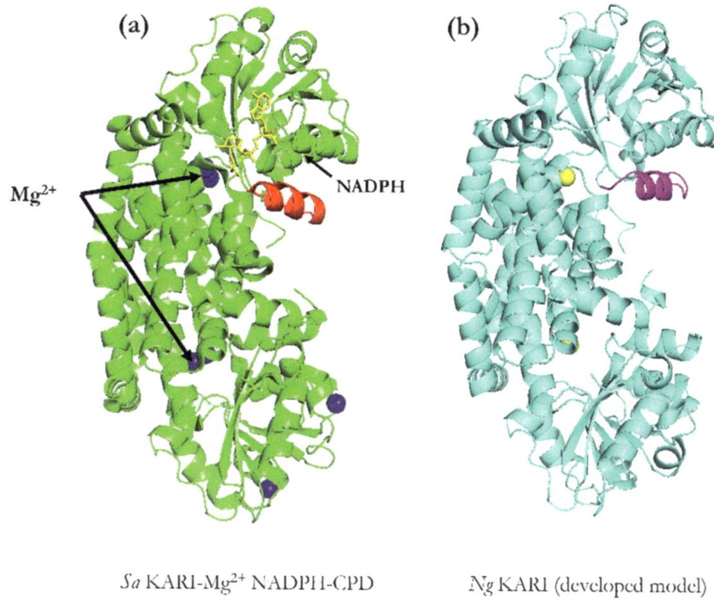

Figure 5.
Comparison of the crystal structure of the Ng KARI (model) with Sa KARI-Mg^{2+}-NADPH-CPD complex. (a) Mg^{2+} ions (blue), and NADPH (red) are shown, respectively, as spheres and sticks. In (b) the Mg^{2+} ions (yellow) are drawn as spheres. The residues colored in red in Sa KARI (i.e. residues 131–145) and magenta in Ng KARI (i.e. residues 130–144) have different orientations in the two enzymes, probably due to the binding of NADPH.

comparison of the N-terminal section of *Ng* KARI with the *Sa* KARI shows that they are some prominent structural differences, particularly in the region from *Ng* KARI as illustrated in **Figure 5**.

The overall fold of the *Ng* KARI resembles that of the *Sa* KARI-NADP(H) complex. No significant domain movements are observed between these two enzymes apart from a change in orientation of the polypeptide associated with the NADP(H) binding site. KARIs from class I differ in their quaternary structures by being dimeric like *Ng* KARI, *Sa* KARI, and KARI from *Mycobacterium tuberculosis* (*Mt* KARI), while others like KARI from *Campylobacter jejuni* (*Cj* KARI) are dodecameric. In their respective active sites, there are two differences between *Ng* KARI and *Sa* KARI, i.e., G100/A106 and L103/ F109. These differences are conserved between *Ng* KARI and *Mt* KARI, G100/G104, L103/L107, with G130/G129. The catalytic residue E230 and Mg^{2+} ligands are highly conserved between all tested pathogens.

3.4 KARI structure analysis

The KARI crystal structure is an asymmetric dimer. This latter is formed by one protomer in the holo-form due to the cofactors (Mg^{2+} and NADP(H)) binding, while the other is in the apo-form. As described previously for similar KARI enzymes, the dimerization is crucial for the construction of the active site, which is formed by some regions of the N-terminal domain and C-terminal domain of one subunit and the C-domain of the other subunit in the dimer. This arrangement is shared by other KARIs from other bacteria.

The KARI enzyme is composed of two distinct domains, the N-terminal (1–181) and C-terminal (182–327). The N-terminal domain, composed of alpha helix and beta sheets, harbor the NADPH-binding domain ilvN (14–177), with the binding sites for NADP (R48 and S52), while the catalytic domain ilvC is present in the C-terminal domain (183–326). The metal binding sites are present in both N-terminal and C-terminal domains (N39, V70, K71, and A73), and (D190 and E194), respectively. The structure of KARI binds four Mg^{2+} ions in the active sites and five Mg^{2+} on the surface of the protein.

A high electron density is shown in two locations deep inside the active site of KARI. This density is ascribed to magnesium ions coordinated differently to the structure. The first Mg^{2+} ion (Mg^{2+} (I)) is coordinated by the side chains of two residues (D188 and E192), and four water molecules, while the second Mg^{2+}(II) is coordinated by the side chains of D188, E224 and E228, in addition to three water molecules. The metal ligands adopt an octahedron coordination geometry, with distances varying between 2.0 and 2.1 A between the metal and its ligand. The average B-factors for Mg^{2+}(I) and Mg^{2+}(II) are 11.5 Å2 and 10 Å2, respectively, supporting a highly ordered structure in this region of KARI [26].

Because of the absence of crystal structures of KARI from *N. gonorrhoeae*, the structure analysis is based on similar structure for close organisms having similar amino acid sequences. Based on the crystal structure of Mg KARI, the active site pocket and thus the magnesium ions are exposed to the solvent, allowing ready access to the substrates, the NADPH, or an inhibitor able to prevent their binding to the structure. The expected binding site for NADPH includes residues from Y22 to G26. All these residues are solvent accessible, hence the residue S24 seems to be the main entrance to the active site. Thus, the designed inhibitors should be designed that target this surface with metal coordination.

4. Conclusion

Increasing concerns associated with overusing antibiotics in animals and humans make it urgent to find new alternatives for treating bacterial infections and diseases. BCAA pathways enzymes are promising antimicrobial alternatives being developed as potential drug targets absent in animals and humans. Comparative studies of KARI from different bacteria bestows the idea that this essential enzyme can be targeted for anti-bacterial drug design. Therefore, KARI is considered a good target, due to a non-homologous protein in comparison with human proteins, and its targeting will be safe for humans. In this review, we assess the presence of KARI in most human pathogens, especially the ESKAPE group, due to its high antibiotic-resistance causing severe infections.

Since the 3D structure for KARI from *N. gonorrhoeae* was nonreported yet, a model of this enzyme was produced using the Swiss model. Indeed, the *Ng* KARI was modeled in silico based on X-ray crystallography structure for *Sa* KARI, used as a template. It was evaluated that cofactors ligands (Mg^{2+} and NADPH) were conserved among human bacterial pathogens. Upon the binding of these cofactors, KARI adapts a different conformation allowing the substrate binding and catalysis, while the active site adapt to a closed state.

Competitive inhibitors, targeting the active site are promoting drugs for the growth inhibition of pathogens. However, the NADPH binding site and the active site are highly conserved among bacteria, including the gut microbiome. In fact, a growing number of studies have shown that antibiotics can result in microbial dysbiosis, due to their broad-spectrum activities, when subsets of commensal microbes will be indiscriminately killed or inhibited. Notably, different antibiotics or their combinations have different antimicrobial spectra and will result in different damages to the microbiome. The disruption of gut microbiota contributes to numerous diseases, including diabetes, obesity, autism, and superinfection in critically ill patients.

Under normal physiological conditions, the microbiota maintains a homeostatic state. It also plays a crucial role in many aspects of physiological processes, including maintaining the integrity of the gut mucosal barrier, promoting the development of the immune system, and protecting against enteric pathogens. Inappropriate antibiotics impact host immunity by altering the bacterial metabolites and the signals transmitted from gut microbiota to the host (intestinal epithelial cells and intestinal immune cells).

Because antibiotic administration elicits many side effects, restriction of the overuse of antibiotics is imperative. However, it is unrealistic to completely abandon antibiotics in clinical practice, especially for patients with severe infections. Therefore, safe strategies should be proposed to attenuate and/or avoid antibiotic-induced microbial dysbiosis and gut microbiome disruption. Firstly, intravenous administration of KARI's inhibitors drugs (or adjuvant) may avoid the gut flora alteration. The adjuvant administration can be followed by the administration of PRRs agonist, or probiotics. Indeed, the probiotic intervention is able to reduce the antibiotic-associated diarrhea [27]. A recent study suggested that co-administration of probiotics and antibiotics prevents *C. difficile* infection in patients receiving antibiotics [28]. On the other hand, gut microbiota transplantation is a new strategy able to control intestinal inflammation and restore the intestinal homeostasis.

KARI's inhibitors remain a good alternative for external treatment for dermatological infections like staphylococcal skin infections in deep wounds. The external application or the intravenous administration of the drug will avoid the alteration of gut flora. Even with need for an oral administration of these drugs, the disorder of gut flora will be partial, due to the high population density of a healthy microbiome, compared to pathogens. Therefore, probiotics can help to maintain the gut flora in sufficient density to maintain the gut mucosal barrier.

Moreover, KARI is an attractive target for the development of new biocides. Some tested KARI's inhibitors inhibit the enzyme in the nanomolar range [29]. Furthermore, the study of KARI-expression during bacterial host-infection may confer new insight on the importance of these targets in the pathogen metabolism and growth. The investigation of the effect of potent KARI's inhibitors on pathogen growth in the presence or not of appropriate antibiotic allow further progress toward the understanding of the inhibitor's effect on pathogen and host-homeostasis, and the development of new inhibitors that specifically target KARIs in pathogenic processes.

Conflict of interest

The authors declare no conflict of interest.

Author details

Emna Rigane and Susu M. Zughaier*
Department of Basic Medical Sciences, College of Medicine, QU Health, Qatar University, Doha, Qatar

*Address all correspondence to: szughaier@qu.edu.qa

References

[1] Wun SJ, Johnson LA, You L, McGeary RP, Brueck T, Schenk G, et al. Inhibition studies of ketol-acid reductoisomerase from pathogenic microorganisms. Archives of Biochemistry and Biophysics. 2020;**692**:108516

[2] Ey L, Pc A, Jd K. Epidemiology, treatments, and vaccine development for antimicrobial-resistant *Neisseria gonorrhoeae*: Current strategies and future directions. Drugs. Jul 2021;**81**:1153-1169. DOI: 10.1007/s40265-021-01530-0

[3] Unemo M, Nicholas RA. Emergence of multidrug-resistant, extensively drug-resistant and untreatable gonorrhea. Future Microbiology. 2012;7:1401-1422

[4] Quillin SJ, Seifert HS. *Neisseria gonorrhoeae* host-adaptation and pathogenesis. Nature Reviews. Microbiology. 2018;**16**:226-240

[5] Voter AF, Callaghan MM, Tippana R, Myong S, Dillard JP, Keck JL. Antigenic variation in *Neisseria gonorrhoeae* occurs independently of RecQ-mediated unwinding of the pilE G quadruplex. Journal of Bacteriology. 2020;**202**:e00607-e00619

[6] Zughaier SM, Kandler JL, Shafer WM. *Neisseria gonorrhoeae* modulates iron-limiting innate immune defenses in macrophages. PLoS One. 2014;**9**:e87688

[7] Lutz AR. Screening forasymptomatic extragenital *Gonorrhoea* and *Chlamydia* in men who have sex with men: Significance, recommendations, and options for overcoming barriers to testing. LGBT Health. 2015;**2**:27-34

[8] Workowski KA, Bachmann LH, Chan PA, Johnston CM, Muzny CA, Park I, et al. Sexually transmitted infections treatment guidelines, 2021. MMWR - Recommendations and Reports. 2021;**70**:1-187

[9] Gonorrhea in women: symptoms, diagnosis, causes, and treatment. Flohealth - 1 Mob Prod Women's Health. 2022. Available from: https://flo.health/menstrual-cycle/sex/stis/gonorrhea-in-women [Accessed: September 6, 2022].

[10] Gonorrhoea - Symptoms. NhsUk 2018. 2022. Available from: https://www.nhs.uk/conditions/gonorrhoea/symptoms/ [Accessed: September 6, 2022]

[11] Gonorrhea: Causes & Symptoms. Clevel Clin. 2022. Available from: https://my.clevelandclinic.org/health/diseases/4217-gonorrhea [Accessed: September 6, 2022].

[12] Whelan J, Abbing-Karahagopian V, Serino L, Unemo M. Gonorrhoea: A systematic review of prevalence reporting globally. BMC Infectious Diseases. 2021;**21**:1152

[13] Unemo M, Shafer WM. Antimicrobial resistance in *Neisseria gonorrhoeae* in the 21st century: Past, evolution, and future. Clinical Microbiology Reviews. 2014;**27**:587-613

[14] Huband MD, Bradford PA, Otterson LG, Basarab GS, Kutschke AC, Giacobbe RA, et al. In Vitro antibacterial activity of AZD0914, a new Spiropyrimidinetrione DNA Gyrase/Topoisomerase inhibitor with potent activity against Gram-Positive, fastidious Gram-Negative, and atypical bacteria | Antimicrobial Agents and Chemotherapy. Jan 2015;**59**(1):467-474

[15] Abrams AJ, Trees DL. Genomic sequencing of *Neisseria gonorrhoeae*

to respond to the urgent threat of antimicrobial-resistant gonorrhea. Pathogens and Disease. Jun 2017;**75**(4): ftx041. Available from: https:// DOI org/10.1093/femspd/ftx041

[16] Morse SA, Johnson SR, Biddle JW, Roberts MC. High-level tetracycline resistance in *Neisseria gonorrhoeae* is result of acquisition of streptococcal tetM determinant. Antimicrobial Agents and Chemotherapy. 1986;**30**:664-670

[17] Morya VK, Kumari S, Kim E. Virtual screening and evaluation of Ketol-acid Reducto-Isomerase (KARI) as a putative drug target for Aspergillosis. Clinical Proteomics. 2012;**9**:1

[18] Lin X, Kurz JL, Patel KM, Wun SJ, Hussein WM, Lonhienne T, et al. Discovery of a pyrimidinedione derivative with potent inhibitory activity against *mycobacterium tuberculosis* Ketol-acid Reductoisomerase. Angew Chem Weinheim Bergstr Ger. 2021;**27**:3130-3141

[19] Wang Y, Liu S, Yin X, Yu D, Xie X, Huang B. Functional analysis of Keto-acid Reductoisomerase ILVC in the entomopathogenic fungus *Metarhizium robertsii*. Journal of Fungi. 2021;**7**:737

[20] Krishna VS, Zheng S, Rekha EM, Nallangi R, Sai Prasad DV, George SE, et al. Design and development of ((4-methoxyphenyl)carbamoyl) (5-(5-nitrothiophen-2-yl)-1,3,4-thiadiazol-2-yl)amide analogues as *mycobacterium tuberculosis* ketol-acid reductoisomerase inhibitors. European Journal of Medicinal Chemistry. 2020;**193**:112178

[21] Clustal W, Clustal X version 2.0 | Bioinformatics | Oxford Academic. 2022. Available from: https:// academic.oup.com/bioinformatics/ article/23/21/2947/371686 [Accessed: August 21, 2022]

[22] Kumar S, Nei M, Dudley J, Tamura K. MEGA: A biologist-centric software for evolutionary analysis of DNA and protein sequences. Briefings in Bioinformatics. 2008;**9**:299-306

[23] DeLano WL. Pymol: An open-source molecular graphics tool. CCP4 Newsl Protein Crystallography. 2002;**40**:82-92

[24] Chen C-Y, Ko T-P, Lin K-F, Lin B-L, Huang C-H, Chiang C-H, et al. NADH/NADPH bi-cofactor-utilizing and thermoactive ketol-acid reductoisomerase from *Sulfolobus acidocaldarius*. Scientific Reports. 2018;**8**:7176

[25] Kim G, Shin D, Lee S, Yun J, Lee S. Crystal structure of IlvC, a Ketol-acid Reductoisomerase, from *streptococcus Pneumoniae*. Crystals. 2019;**9**:551

[26] Lv Y, Kandale A, Wun SJ, McGeary RP, Williams SJ, Kobe B, et al. Crystal structure of *mycobacterium tuberculosis* ketol-acid reductoisomerase at 1.0 Å resolution – A potential target for anti-tuberculosis drug discovery. The FEBS Journal. 2016;**283**:1184-1196

[27] Zhang S, Chen D-C. Facing a new challenge: The adverse effects of antibiotics on gut microbiota and host immunity. Chinese Medical Journal. 2019;**132**:1135-1138

[28] Goldenberg JZ, Mertz D, Johnston BC. Probiotics to prevent *Clostridium difficile* infection in patients receiving antibiotics. JAMA. 2018;**320**:499

[29] Bayaraa T, Kurz JL, Patel KM, Hussein WM, Bilyj JK, West NP, et al. Discovery, synthesis and evaluation of a novel ketol-acid reductoisomerase inhibitor. Angew Chem Weinheim Bergstr Ger. 2020;**26**(41):8958-8968